Praise for BLACK BELT FITNESS FOR LIFE

"There's something to martial arts and especially the way Grandmaster Kang teaches it that addresses not just the body and fitness, but addresses the mind and addresses your approach to life."

—from the foreword by Michael Imperioli, award-winning actor

"In these pages you will find the essence of Grandmaster Kang's teachings, philosophy and workout programs, all of which are transformative—not only from a physical standpoint, but more importantly, from a mental standpoint."

—Andrew J. Federici, award-winning Internet executive

"I've learned the importance of stretching and exercising on a regular basis from my experience as a healthcare professional for the last 17 years. Grandmaster Kang's fitness regiment is not only a great way to stay in shape but can also help prevent injuries, especially as we age." —Dr. John R. Gehnrich D.C.

"As someone who enjoys the physical nature of Taekwondo, as well as triathlons, mountaineering and 24 hour endurance races, Grandmaster Kang has helped me strengthen not only my body but my mental capacity as well. It is only once you have experienced the guidance in life that he brings that you start to learn what you are really capable of. From a renowned lineage in the martial arts, he has the unique ability to bring out the best in you."

—Alexander (Alf) Garner, CEO Faber Global North America

"The T. Kang Taekwondo website states 'A tradition of excellence since 1969'; this is a rare truth in today's hyped-up social media era. Grandmaster Kang runs an outstanding program that has truly benefited both me and my family. I'm less stressed and more focused at work, and my kids have become more attentive and successful at school and in sports. Training under Grandmaster Kang as a family and earning our black belts has been an exceedingly rewarding experience."

—Robert Vecchio, Ph.D., P.E., CEO/Principal Lucius Pitkin, Inc.

BLACK BELT FITNESS FOR LIFE

A 7-WEEK PLAN TO ACHIEVE LIFELONG WELLNESS

Grandmaster **TAE SUN KANG**

with a foreword by **MICHAEL IMPERIOLI**

TUTTLE Publishing

Tokyo | Rutland, Vermont | Singapore

Please note that the publisher and author of this instructional book are NOT RESPONSIBLE in any manner whatsoever for any injury that may result from practicing the techniques and/or following the instructions given within. Martial arts training can be dangerous—both to you and to others—if not practiced safely. If you're in doubt as to how to proceed or whether your practice is safe, consult with a trained martial arts teacher before beginning. Since the physical activities described herein may be too strenuous in nature for some readers, it is also essential that a physician be consulted prior to training.

The Tuttle Story:
"Books to Span the East and West"

Many people are surprised to learn that the world's leading publisher of books on Asia had humble beginnings in the tiny American state of Vermont. The company's founder, Charles E. Tuttle, belonged to a New England family steeped in publishing.

Immediately after WWII, Tuttle served in Tokyo under General Douglas MacArthur and was tasked with reviving the Japanese publishing industry. He later founded the Charles E. Tuttle Publishing Company, which thrives today as one of the world's leading independent publishers.

Though a westerner, Tuttle was hugely instrumental in bringing a knowledge of Japan and Asia to a world hungry for information about the East. By the time of his death in 1993, Tuttle had published over 6,000 books on Asian culture, history and art—a legacy honored by the Japanese emperor with the "Order of the Sacred Treasure," the highest tribute Japan can bestow upon a non-Japanese.

With a backlist of 1,500 titles, Tuttle Publishing is more active today than at any time in its past—inspired by Charles Tuttle's core mission to publish fine books to span the East and West and provide a greater understanding of each.

Published by Tuttle Publishing, an imprint of Periplus Editions (HK) Ltd.

www.tuttlepublishing.com

Library of Congress Cataloging-in-Publication Data
Kang, Tae Sun.
  Black belt fitness for life : a 7-week plan to achieve lifelong wellness / Grandmaster Tae Sun Kang, with a foreword by Michael Imperioli.
    pages cm
  ISBN 978-0-8048-4374-4 (paperback -- ISBN 978-1-4629-1524-8 (ebook) 1. Black belt fitness for life I. Title.
                2014030058

ISBN 978-0-8048-4374-4

First edition
19 18 17 16 15   5 4 3 2 1   1505MP
Printed in Singapore

Front Cover and Interior Photography by Claire Jones
Back Cover Photography by Henry Leutwyler

Distributed by

North America, Latin America & Europe
364 Innovation Drive
North Clarendon, VT 05759-9436 U.S.A.
Tel: (802) 773-8930; Fax: (802) 773-6993
info@tuttlepublishing.com; www.tuttlepublishing.com

Japan
Tuttle Publishing
Yaekari Building, 3rd Floor
5-4-12 Osaki, Shinagawa-ku, Tokyo 141 0032
Tel: (81) 3 5437-0171; Fax: (81) 3 5437-0755
sales@tuttle.co.jp; www.tuttle.co.jp

Asia Pacific
Tuttle Publishing
Berkeley Books Pte. Ltd.
61 Tai Seng Avenue #02-12, Singapore 534167
Tel: (65) 6280-1330; Fax: (65) 6280-6290
inquiries@periplus.com.sg; www.periplus.com

Indonesia
PT Java Books Indonesia
Jl. Rawa Gelam IV No. 9
Kawasan Industri Pulogadung, Jakarta 13930
Tel: (62) 21 4682-1088; Fax: (62) 21 461-0206
crm@periplus.co.id; www.periplus.com

TUTTLE PUBLISHING® is a registered trademark of Tuttle Publishing, a division of Periplus Editions (HK) Ltd.

Contents

Foreword *by Michael Imperioli*... 7

Editor's Note *by Andrew J. Federici* 9

CHAPTER 1

Finding the Will—The Story of Grandmaster Tae Sun Kang 11

CHAPTER 2

Jump Start.. 19

CHAPTER 3

Finding the Fountain of Youth... 29

    Developing Confidence with the Right Attitude....................................... 34

CHAPTER 4

Developing Confidence through the Tenets of Taekwondo....................... 37

    A Message for Parents 42

CHAPTER 5

Exercise and Food Plan for Life.. 47

    Combined Dynamic Stretching 51

    White Belt Beginner Level (Week One)... 57

    Yellow Belt Beginner Level (Week Two).. 74

    Green Belt Intermediate Level (Week Three)... 78

    Blue Belt Intermediate Level (Week Four)... 97

    Brown Belt Advanced Level (Week Five) 100

Red Belt Advanced Level (Week Six) 126

Black Belt Advanced Level (Week Seven and Beyond) 129

Forms for Meditation 136

Testimonials 145

CHAPTER 6

Self-Defense 149

Self-Defense Techniques 152

Conclusion 159

Foreword

by Michael Imperioli

My children started doing Taekwondo with Grandmaster Tae Sun Kang about six months before I started in 2003. I had been on the road, working on a couple of movies—two shootings back to back from the end of the summer until November. I returned to New York and was really out of shape. I was smoking cigarettes a lot, drinking too much, and not eating correctly. I hadn't been exercising for a long time—in fact, many years—and I was really scared. I actually started with a couple of private lessons with Grandmaster because the idea of jumping right into the class with other students was a little bit frightening to me.

I had tried joining gyms, and I joined an aerobics-type class once, but I never stuck to anything as far as fitness programs went. I was afraid that I would eventually give up on this too, to be honest. I was afraid that I couldn't hack it. I felt too old, too out of shape.

What got me through were a couple of things. The first thing was Grandmaster Kang—his integrity, and his genuine interest in the well-being of his students. He instilled in me the basics of Taekwondo, teaching me the basic kicks and some of the simpler stretches. He really instilled in me the idea that if I just stuck with it, then I would make some progress. Nothing's going to happen if I didn't come regularly. Because I was still smoking and I really wasn't healthy, it was hard getting through these early workouts. But I remember saying to myself, "just get to the end, don't quit." I never had to stop a workout because of low endurance. I've gotten injured a little here and there and I had to stop taking classes for that, but other than those times, I've always made it through a class. I never said, "that's it, I give up!"

There's something to martial arts, and especially the way Grandmaster Kang teaches it, that addresses not just the body and fitness, but also the mind and your approach to life. The tenets that he promotes—courtesy, integrity, self-control, perseverance, indomitable spirit—these things are very present in his teaching, and they're very important elements.

I was taken aback by the formality of bowing and calling everyone "sir" because I had never been in an atmosphere where you did that. I mean, I'm polite, as polite as anyone else, I would say. But it was a little off-putting at first and I was a little reluctant; I thought it was kind of strange, but now I really appreciate it. I feel it creates a very level playing field among students—we're all equals. Whatever belt level we have, we still bow to each other. I bow to white belts because I have respect for their choice to come here.

To bow to your Grandmaster and to your instructors and to the flags, it gives a certain respect to these things and to the discipline. The respect you give it is that firstly, it may save your life one day, or the life of a loved one, or the life of a stranger on the street, because maybe you'll have to defend them against someone who's trying to do some serious harm. And it may save your life by the way that it's going to keep you healthy, it's going extend your life and keep your family healthy. It's not just a trendy thing that's going to get you six pack abs, although you can certainly achieve that if you try.

I think the respect shown at Grandmaster's studio really separates this place from the outside world, and it's not just another workout. It's something that's beneficial to mind, body, and spirit. I find myself calling people "sir" in life, too. And I think that's all right. People appreciate that. I call people "sir" and "ma'am" all the time. We're all human beings—if you show me respect and I show you respect, things will go a lot smoother in the world.

Editor's Note

by Andrew J. Federici

I met Grandmaster Kang in the summer of 2006. I had just started working for MTV, and after watching a film about Taekwondo, I decided to fulfill a childhood dream of learning a martial art.

After years of on-again, off-again yoga, random visits to the gym, and no consistent exercise regime, I walked into Grandmaster's elegant studio in TriBeCa and found there a lifelong friend, mentor, teacher, and great source of happiness.

In my media career I had the chance to work with various life improvement experts, including some in the fitness arena. And while many were talented, few exuded the kind of warmth, authenticity, and practical wisdom of Grandmaster Kang.

In my time studying with Grandmaster, from White Belt all the way to 2nd Dan Black Belt, I found solace, a special place where worries melted away as we studied ancient forms, sparred against each other, and attempted harder and harder techniques, constantly stretching our minds and bodies to greater heights.

In studying with Grandmaster Kang, I soon realized that his style of teaching, motivation, authenticity, and vision was unique and that it needed to be shared on a wider scale. It was then that the idea of this book was born.

In these pages you will find the essence of Grandmaster's teachings, philosophy, and workout programs, all of which are transformative, not only from a physical standpoint, but more importantly from a mental standpoint.

Through practice of these routines you will find your physique improved, your concentration better, you will focus more clearly on the important things in your life, and you will find the strength to overcome any challenge.

This is what I gained from studying with Grandmaster Kang and through this book, you can too!

Andrew J. Federici
T. Kang Taekwondo student, 2nd Dan Black Belt

Finding the Will—The Story of Grandmaster Tae Sun Kang

I know what it's like to be out of shape, to be unhappy because of the way you look or feel. If you're reading this book and you feel the same way, you're not alone. Over the years, I've helped thousands of people get into the best shape of their lives mentally and physically—and I can do the same for you. Let me teach you a method and mindset that can turn exercise into an enjoyable part of your life instead of a chore.

In the end, it's not an exercise regimen or diet that will change you, it's your attitude that will change you. Give me a chance to be your personal coach to guide you through this journey to change your attitude and become a healthier, more confident, and happier person.

If it wasn't for Taekwondo, I wouldn't be writing this book. Like many of you, I've had my share of ups and downs, sleepless nights caused by stress, doubt, and fear of failure. I can honestly say Taekwondo has saved my mental, physical, and spiritual health.

I've been in the fitness industry since I was a teenager and have been a practitioner of the martial arts for over 40 years. I learned from watching my father, Grandmaster Suh Chong Kang. During summers when most of my friends were away at camp or out all day playing sports or hanging out, I was stuck at the Do Jang (Taekwondo school) in Brooklyn, NY. My father held a very high position in the Taekwondo community, and because of this, he was frequently out of town at seminars, tournaments, and belt tests. It was up to me and my two older brothers to run his studio. I was only 13 when he put me to work. At 16, my older brothers went off to college and I had to run it by myself. After school, I'd rush to the studio, teach classes, and do my homework when I had any free time. After closing up, I'd get home at 11 pm, have dinner, and finish the rest of my homework. Despite this, I still had good grades. When the teenagers I teach today complain about all the school work they have, I have to laugh. I wish when I was their age all I had to worry about was homework.

Having reached my full height at 13 years old, I told students I was really 18. Back then, the martial arts was all about who was the toughest and the best fighter. People came in to learn how to fight, not stay in shape. The only way these people would take me seriously as an instructor was if they thought I was older than I really was. It's one thing to tell people you're 18 when you're only 13, but it's another thing altogether to act like you are. Before taking over the responsibility of running my father's school, I was a typical teenager. Every other word that came out of my mouth was a four-letter word. But when I had people looking up to me as a role model and really respecting me—even people who were old enough to be my parents—I realized that I had to behave a certain way. Even the top instructors under me never knew I was only a few years older than them.

I have to admit; I was not happy at this point in my life. Miserable would be the right word. Believe it or not, I actually hated teaching Taekwondo then. I hated that I had no choice about whether or not I wanted to run my father's school. At 18, when I decided to go to college and pursue my own goals, I looked at every option other than Taekwondo. I never wanted to teach it again or run a school. The main reason for that was my father.

When Michael Jackson died, I realized I had a lot in common with him. I learned he hated his father because his father took away his childhood and forced him to work. Not only that, he was physically and emotionally abusive. The only difference between his father and mine is that my father didn't physically abuse any of us. And thank goodness! The man was capable of killing someone with a single punch or kick.

In Korea, he was the head instructor of the Korean Military Intelligence Agency and the commanding instructor for the entire Korean army. Part of his job was interrogating North Korean prisoners of war. He used to routinely terrify grown men! Having worked for the Korean Military Intelligence Agency, he knew how to scare people and get in their heads.

People that know him have nothing but praise for him. To them, not only was he a great Taekwondo instructor, but also a great person. He would go out of his way to help people. What these people didn't see is the side of him when he drank. My father was an alcoholic. He drank every night and every time he got drunk, he turned into a completely different person. I saw, from a very young age, the destructive power of alcohol. Every night, from dinner until 4 am in the morning, my parents would fight. That sounds like an exaggeration but it was the truth. I can't remember even one single time they didn't fight all night. I remember telling my mom to divorce my father. I told her this man was no good for her. Can you imagine that, a son telling his mom to get a divorce?

When he got drunk every night, I could see the fury in his eyes. The smallest things set him off. If the dinner wasn't to his liking, he'd go into a rage. Like I said, he never physically abused us, but the fear of being physically abused was always present. And let me tell you, when he stared at you with his angry eyes, I don't care how tough you are, it was scary! I'd stay up all night to make sure he didn't hurt anyone. He'd go to sleep around 4 am and only when I knew he was asleep did I feel safe enough to go to sleep.

Later on, I started dating the woman who would become my wife. She was the only person I could talk to about my father, but she was a student at the school and only saw the sober, instructor side of my father. She came over one night and witnessed firsthand what I had to deal with every night. I was sitting on the couch with her when my father went into another rage—he was seething with anger. I whispered to Cristina to not make a noise and just sit there as quietly as she could. She looked terrified. I could see she was doing everything she could to not upset him, she didn't even want to make eye contact with him. As soon as my father fell asleep, she ran out the door and told me she never wanted to come back.

My parents later separated and my mother and second oldest brother moved out West to Seattle. My oldest brother was away at college. I was the only one patient enough to stay with my father. Every morning, when he was sober, he acted like nothing had happened. It was just like living with Dr. Jekyll and Mr. Hyde. Living with someone like that took a toll on me physically, emotionally, and mentally. And eventually even my patience wore out. I couldn't afford a place on my own, so I moved in with Cristina's family until I was able to get my own place.

It was tough enough dealing with my father when he was drunk, but it was no picnic to live with him when he was sober, either. All I wanted was what every kid wants—to feel loved and secure, to know that your father supports you and cares for you. I never had that from him, nor did any of my brothers. We never even had one word of encouragement or guidance from him. It wasn't like he was incapable of showing warmth and love. To his friends and colleagues, he was amazingly kind. He treated them better than he did his own family.

Most parents will break their backs working so they can give their kids the life they never had. It was the reverse scenario with me. My parents made me work like a dog so they could live the life they wanted to live. During high school, I had to have early dismissal every day just so I could get to the Taekwondo school on time to teach. My older brothers left as soon as they had the chance, and never came back. I can't blame them for that, I think I would've done the same if I had the chance. I was the youngest and only one left, so I had the burden of running the school by myself. My parents used to be gone for days at a time, often on vacation or business, and when they came back, my father would go to the school just to see if it made any money. And if it didn't make enough, he'd get angry. I remember often thinking, "I'm only a teenager and running this big school by myself—what do you expect?!" Imagine how you would feel if your boss made you run a business by yourself and only came into work when it was time to collect the money.

Because my parents were never around, I learned quickly that the only person I could depend on was myself. No matter what happened, I realized the only person that would be there for me, was me. I couldn't depend on my parents, and so it was up to me to run the business, go to school, cook my meals. This is something I still carry with me to this day. I've never once had a personal trainer. When I exercise, the one thing that gets me through a workout is my will power. If I'm lifting weights, I don't even like having someone spot me. I want to push through that last set using sheer will power. Growing up the way I did made me very independent and self-reliant.

Looking back, I can understand why my father was so unaffection-ate with me and my brothers. His father died when he was nine years old and growing up in Korea during times of war was tough. My child-hood didn't feel any different from his. I felt like I grew up without a father. I can still remember my childhood in Korea. Because of the Ko-rean War, poverty was rampant in the countryside where we lived. My mother, my two brothers and I lived in the back of someone's house in a tiny room. It would be the equivalent of living in someone's garage. That one room was our bedroom, living room, and dining room.

My father was never around, but even if he was, it wouldn't have made a difference, because he didn't really care about his family. All we had to eat were soybean sprouts, called *Kongnamul* in Korean. That's all we had, just that and rice every day for every meal. For some meals, the soybean sprouts were pan fried, for others we ate it as a soup or steamed. But that was literally our only option when it came to food.

When things got really bad, I went from house to house to beg for food. My older brothers were too embarrassed to do it, so I had to. It wasn't like the families around us were doing any better. We were all living in poverty. I wonder if children today realize how lucky they are. They have their own rooms, video games, iPhones and iPods, clothes they don't have to share with siblings, meals any time they want. They take all of these things for granted. The family whose house we lived in had a TV, and they'd let us watch it for one hour a week. Watching that TV for that one hour was a luxury for me.

I believe every parent has a choice in how to raise their kids. If they were raised by unloving, abusive parents, they could raise their kids the same way, without any love. Or they can do the opposite and shower them with love. One time I was with my daughter Sofia, who was 3 at the time, at a restaurant and I remember three older women kept look-ing over at us from their table. I wondered why they kept looking over constantly. When we finished and were leaving, they came up to me and told me they've never seen a father show so much love and atten-tion to a child before. They said I must have had a really good role model growing up. In a way, they were right. My father made me realize that I never wanted to treat my kids the way he treated his. I wish I didn't have to learn that way, I wish he could have shown us even just a fraction of the good he's shown other people. It's unfortunate, but in life, sometimes pain is our best teacher.

Even through all that, what kept me sane and focused was Taekwondo. I hated teaching it and running the school, but I've always loved practicing Taekwondo. It was the only thing that made me feel good. I was chubby growing up and my brothers used to call me "fat boy" all the time, so I loved that doing Taekwondo helped me lose weight and feel confident about myself. No matter how bad things got because of my father, when I did Taekwondo, it was always a great stress reliever. It made me feel like I could handle whatever came next. I figured I could always practice Taekwondo on my own—I didn't need to practice it at my father's school—so even though I loved training, I was still looking for a way out of running my father's school.

After I graduated high school, I enrolled at an engineering college, Polytechnic University (now NYU Polytechnic), but after a couple of months, I had to drop all my classes. Even though I was taking a full semester's load of classes, my father didn't care. He still made me run the school fulltime without anyone to assist me. That's how it was for me during my high school years too. My father never paid any interest in how I did at school. All that mattered was that I taught the classes and made money for him. During my first semester at college, I'd only have an hour a day to study for six classes. Some days, the only time I had to do homework was on the train! So to make my schedule easier, I enrolled at two other local colleges in New York and I did very well but it wasn't what I was looking for. One of my dreams was to be an actor, so I pursued that. I enrolled in acting school at the American Academy of Dramatic Arts and really learned about myself there.

I became friends with the other students and they used to complain all the time about work. Most of them waited tables and hated their jobs, they hated how people treated them. I thought about my own job situation. At the Taekwondo school, everyone called me "sir" and treated not only me with respect, but their fellow students as well. I realized it wasn't the teaching and running the school aspect that I hated. It was teaching and running the school for my father.

I thought about opening my own school and just separating from my father, but I saw the potential of my father's school. My father taught the same class every time, he placed a heavy emphasis on basics, but I could see the students were getting bored. He didn't have the creativity I had in teaching different types of classes. At 22, I made a deal with him and bought the business from him. Part of the terms of the deal was that I would pay off his credit card debt and pay for his living expenses for 20 years. This included paying his rent and bills. It basically let him retire a lot earlier than he would have. When I first offered him a deal to buy his school, he laughed. He didn't take me seriously and he laughed every time I asked him. But I was persistent and after a year, he finally gave in. The school was mine to run my own way.

People assume he just gave me the school for all the years of working for him for no pay. I wish that was the case! Anything related to tuition or test fees went to my father, but he let me make money from seminars and private lessons. On Saturdays after the last class, I'd do a board-breaking seminar or a sparring seminar or special kicking seminar. I'd experiment with classes. I'd teach a cardio kickboxing class or a stretching class or a body-toning class. This is how a lot of my classes were developed. These classes became so popular, that when I took over the school, I incorporated them into the curriculum. In fact, this method of teaching specialized classes—classes where you work on a specific aspect of Taekwondo, be it basics or kicking or hitting the bag or working on fitness, like cardio, strengthening, and stretching—became so effective that many of my former students who went on to open their own studios used my method of teaching. New students, especially children, often ask me: "Are you a grandmaster because you can beat up anybody and you were a champion in tournaments and you're not intimidated by anyone?"

My answer to them is always, "No, that's not why I'm a grandmaster."

Grandmaster is really a teaching title, like a professor, but in many ways it's a bit more. You can almost say that I'm a teacher of teachers (or professors). It's a title that takes more than a few decades to achieve— it usually requires a lifetime of dedication.

A grandmaster's expertise should go beyond teaching individuals just martial arts skills.

A grandmaster should be able to get into the minds of the students.

A grandmaster should be able to teach them how to develop a higher level of integrity, humility, self awareness, and confidence.

A grandmaster is a teacher who is not selfish, but willing to share his life's hard work, and able to pave an easier and clearer path where others can follow and learn to be their personal best.

Finally, a grandmaster is one who can express his true level of confidence by making his ultimate goal helping others to develop and even surpass himself.

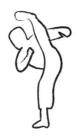

Jump Start

There are many books out there that advocate weight training and dieting for a short period of time—4, 8, 12 weeks, etc. These books show incredible transformations of the body through before and after pictures. How many people do you know, or can think of, that tried one of these workouts or diets and went through an extreme transformation from overweight to shredded and were able to maintain their new bodies? I'm willing to bet not many. What these books don't tell you is that extreme workouts and diets don't work in the long run. To lose that kind of weight in such a short period of time requires extreme physical and mental exertion. Even professional athletes have trouble adjusting from being mostly sedentary during the off-season to getting back into game-day shape. And these are athletes who are still active—retired athletes are a different story! Let's be honest, it's not easy maintaining that kind of discipline after completing one of these workout or diet regimes. They're temporary cures for a permanent situation.

Not only do these extreme workouts and diets not work in the long run, but most of them are based on a short, fixed period of time. If you lost 50 pounds in four weeks, you'll look fantastic. But your internal organs will not reflect how good you look on the surface. When your body goes through such a drastic change in so little time, it wreaks havoc on your internal organs. It's not uncommon for people to experience kidney failure from over-consumption of protein in an attempt to bulk up too quickly. Changes to the body have to be done progressively so the internal organs can adjust to the physiological changes.

You know the story of the tortoise and the hare. Slow and steady wins the race. Gradual progress is the key to losing weight, becoming healthier, and maintaining fitness. Can you picture yourself following one of these intense diets or workout programs for the rest of your life? Even the greatest athletes don't have that kind of discipline. Think of some of your favorite athletes who are now retired. How many of them have been able to maintain the weight they were at when they were active, or even just stay slim? A very small percentage. These athletes have to consume an enormous amount of food daily because they're working out multiple hours a day. Olympic swimmer Michael Phelps reportedly ate 10,000 calories a day while training! That may be an extreme example, but the fact of the matter is once an athlete stops training, the number of calories they burn reduces but their appetite doesn't. The only way they can keep the weight off is if they continue to train like they did during their professional careers. That's a very tough thing to do. That's why my system will work. It's not designed just for people in their prime, it's designed for any age group—and it's something you can do your whole life.

In my 40-plus years of working in the fitness industry and teaching students, I've found that one of the problems with exercise is that people dread it. If most people have a choice whether to exercise or not, most will not. It's not until something happens—like not being able to fit into an old pair of jeans or being told by your doctor that you have high blood pressure or even worse, having a stroke—that they realize exercise is the only option. And by then, exercise becomes a chore. I've been exercising all my life, not because I was forced to but because I enjoy it. It's something I look forward to every day. I can help you feel the same way. It's never too late. You might think you have a long road ahead but the sooner you get on that road, the shorter it will seem.

The first thing you have to do is be selfish. Now I don't mean drop everything and do whatever you want and go on a wild shopping spree. I mean be selfish when it comes to exercising and taking care of yourself. Some of you might be thinking, "but I have no time!" Do you really have no time? If the only things you're doing are working, sleeping, eating and nothing else, seven days a week, then yes, I believe you when you say you have no time. But usually, you can squeeze in the time. It won't be easy. You might have to make some sacrifices. Maybe you might have to miss some TV time or not go out and socialize one night, or wake up a little earlier or go to sleep later; but I'm certain you can find the time. If you met the person of your dreams and he or she asked you out on a date, would you say you have no time? You'd find a way to make time! You can always make time for something if you really want to. And think about this: the healthier you are, the longer you will live. This is even more of a reason why you should exercise. By finding time to exercise, you'll create more time to enjoy life.

Another problem people have with exercising is that they're too self-conscious about other people's opinions. Or they feel exercising is too difficult. These are great excuses, but if you're not exercising and keeping healthy, who's going to do it for you? I tell my students that their safety is their own personal responsibility. It's the same with your health. If you want to be there for your children, you're going to have to save yourself first, you have to be selfish. If you're on an airplane and there's a sudden loss of cabin pressure, your first instinct might be to put the oxygen masks on your loved ones so you can save them. But how can you help anyone else if you're starving for oxygen? You have to help yourself first in order to help others. Be selfish.

If you have children, by exercising, you'll set a good example. Obesity rates are increasing at an alarming rate for kids in America. I'm sure you care tremendously for your children's health and well-being. And even if you don't exercise, you will still push your child to exercise and eat right. But you have to look at things from their perspective. Your kids are probably wondering why they should exercise if they don't see you exercising? If all you did was sit around the house and play video games, but you told your child not to do the same, they'd think you're a hypocrite. But if you exercise and tell your kids to exercise, they won't question you. We may not be their heroes, but we are their role models. We have a huge influence on our kids, whether they'd like to admit it or not. And that can go both ways. We can be good role models, or bad ones.

My students tell me one of the biggest factors that stop them from going to the gym is feeling unfit and overweight when everyone else is in great shape. If that's the case, don't go to the gym! Maybe the gym is not for you. You have to be able to feel comfortable where you're exercising. Maybe you'll feel more comfortable in the privacy of your home. If you're feeling too self-conscious about what other people think when you're exercising, just remember what Dr. Seuss said: "Those who mind don't matter and those who matter don't mind."

If you're reading this and you don't have any disabilities, you have to realize how fortunate you are. I've discovered something rather interesting in all my years of teaching. The students with the most injuries, the ones who've had knee replacements, hip replacements, back pain, arthritis, you name it—these are the students that train the hardest. My teenage students, on the other hand, sometimes display the least effort in their training. I have to remind them over and over how lucky they are. Not only do they have two arms and two legs, but they have their health. I have to tell them there are people out there whose only wish is to be able to participate in the activities that they take for granted. Think about how badly you would want to just go for a walk if you were paralyzed. The desire to walk in that situation would be overwhelming. Think about that the next time you feel like skipping a workout.

Speaking of teenagers, some of you reading this may be well beyond your teenage years. You might even have children who are in their teens! When you see young people in their prime working out, it can be intimidating. You might think that compared to these fit people, you're at a disadvantage. But you have to remember life is a balance. Everything adds up to a whole. The age of my students range from 3 to 60 plus. Compared to a 5-year-old, the 40-year-old student won't be nearly as flexible. But compared to the 40-year-old, the 5-year-old's focus and concentration will only be a fraction of that of the older student. Everything is a balance. What you might lack in physical strength will be compensated for in mental strength.

I've seen students in their twenties and in great shape who have never had to deal with any adversities, like a major injury. So when they get injured, they don't know how to cope. Often they lose their discipline and gain a ton of weight. They might be strong physically, but weak mentally. However, many of my students in their forties and fifties have had knee surgeries or hip surgeries, so they can't train as intensely as a 20-year-old student. But their determination is so strong. Their bodies might be weak from injuries, but as a consequence their minds become so much stronger. If they're nursing an injury, instead of training harder, they'll train smarter.

I also see a lot of my younger students give up very easily. For them, things come easily—especially fitness—so when they hit a roadblock, they want to quit. With my older students, they have a lot more life experience, so they're more patient and have more perseverance. Never think you're at a disadvantage just because you start late. The majority of my adult students start in their forties and for a lot of them, it's their first time exercising seriously. Everything adds up to a whole.

You also have to remember that getting into shape is not a competition. Well, let me clarify. The only competition you're in is the one with yourself. This is something I tell my students all the time, especially the ones who start Taekwondo later in life. They come in and sometimes see younger beginners who are more flexible than they are. They see these younger students being able to touch their toes in a stretch, or kick higher than them, or punch stronger. They see this and become discouraged. But I tell them that some people, especially the younger ones, are just naturally more flexible. After a year, maybe the younger student's stretch will improve only by a little. But my older students, when they first joined, maybe they couldn't even touch their toes without bending their knees. But after a year, they can reach beyond their toes. So even though the younger student might still be more flexible, the older student has made a greater improvement in their stretching.

If one of your friends loses 20 pounds in 20 days, that's great for your friend, but don't let that be your motivation to lose weight. I'm sure this is something you must've heard from your parents or teachers growing up: "If one of your friends jumped off a bridge, would you?" (What will you do if a friend gained 20 pounds? Are you going to try to match that?)

The temptation is always there to compare ourselves with others; but the problem with this is that too often, we only look at the best parts of someone else's life, whether it's the amount of money they have or how beautiful or in shape they are. We read magazines and compare our appearance to that of a model or celebrity. What if that famous person spent years feeling depressed about how he or she looked, and had plastic surgery? Or that model secretly starved herself because she's unhappy with her body? We don't compare ourselves with that aspect of their lives.

Life isn't a contest or a competition, and getting in shape certainly isn't. If right now you can only reach your knees in a stretch, let that be your starting point, and make it a competition with yourself to reach farther the next month and the month after that. Or if your goal is to eat less, start by eating 100 calories less per day, instead of something drastic like 1,000 calories. Next month, eat 200 calories less per day. Don't worry about the person next to you progressing faster than you.

Now let's imagine that you're the friend that everyone is jealous of because you lost 20 pounds. You'll feel pretty good about yourself, and you should. It's hard work losing any amount of weight. But don't feel too good, don't feel like you're better than everyone else. You should never think you're the best. If you're climbing a mountain and you get to the peak, where's the only place left for you to go? Down. We've seen it happen to the greatest of champions. They get to the top, become complacent, and lose it all. Even after training in Taekwondo for over 40 years, I still don't think of myself as the best. Whether it's being a practitioner of Taekwondo or an instructor, I think of myself not at the peak of the mountain but somewhere near the top. That way, when I look up, I still have a goal to reach for. I never take for granted the skills I've acquired over the years but at the same time, I'm not satisfied either. I'm still hungry to improve. So I still keep practicing and thinking of innovative ways to teach my students.

And when I look down, I see how much progress I've made. When I think I've hit a plateau, I look down and realize that perseverance and an indomitable spirit got me to this stage—and they'll help me get farther up the mountain.

Like most people, I'm not naturally flexible. As a matter of fact, I have to stretch out regularly in order to maintain my flexibility. But that's precisely why I can help you become more flexible than ever before.

Yes, maybe someone who is triple jointed might be able to teach you some exercises to become more flexible, just like someone that was born into a lot of money might be able to teach you how to get rich. But I'd much rather learn how to make money from the person that started with nothing, and stretching from the individual that had to work to become flexible.

I believe there are a handful of top athletes who achieved their status through hard training, and some of them can also teach their craft well. But at the same time, I feel that most of them were gifted individuals who got to where they are through the right guidance.

What I'm trying to say is, don't judge a book by it's cover. There are trainers and there are athletes—the athletes look super and the trainers look so-so. While the athletes worked hard to look and perform at their best, the trainers are the experts in helping the athletes reach their goals.

In martial arts, one of the main points that's always stressed is proper respect, especially respect toward your teacher. Too often, we just look at the final product, and don't pay enough attention to all the dedicated, underlying work. Like after watching a great movie, the audience might comment on how great the acting, the story, or the action was, and then just head out, never waiting to view the credits of the supporting team that made the movie so great.

Imagine that you have to cross a river and there is a bridge to get you to the other side; I want you to think of your teacher/trainer as the bridge that you need to use to get from one point to another, from being out of shape to being in shape. Just because a trainer doesn't have less than five percent body fat and isn't chiseled like someone on the cover of a fitness magazine doesn't mean that this person hasn't got the knowledge and experience to get you into tip-top shape.

In martial arts, it is very common for the instructor to yell at the students in order to command authority or to discipline students (especially younger ones). This rule is also pretty common practice in many households where children don't listen. The parents feel that they must raise their voices, or sometimes even their hands, in order to control their kids.

I have a totally different approach to teaching martial arts. I don't believe that a teacher/trainer has to be on their students' backs, screaming at them all the time, like those exercise or extreme weight-loss infomercials on TV. I'm sure, if you wanted to, you could have joined the Armed Forces or a military bootcamp class, where a drill sergeant screams continuously at you. So what happens when there's no one behind you, pushing you to exercise? Everyone chooses how they want to train, but my philosophy of fitness is to exercise for life.

In this book, my eating or training methods might not seem all that rigorous to some of you, but you're going to be surprised—if you follow my program properly, you will get into the best mental and physical shape of your life!

Our bodies are not made to take too much abuse, especially as we age. We must practice caution when exercising, and even with our eating. Any drastic measures or quick-fix solutions are not the way to go. Exercising and eating properly is a habit you want to engage in every day of your life.

When you last saw yourself in the mirror, were you happy with the way you looked? And right now, are you happy with the way you feel about yourself?

If the answer is *no*, then what are you going to do about it?

Do you want to continue feeling like this? Aren't you sick and tired of how you let yourself go, and how you've come to this point in your life?

For many people, when they feel that the task is too great, they don't even bother to attempt it. That's often the case when it comes to getting into shape. People often feel that they are fighting a losing battle, and admit defeat before the battle even begins.

I'm sure all of you know the progression of a child's development. In the beginning, they can hardly move or sit up; then they learn to roll, then they start to crawl; then, to everyone's amazement, they take their first steps.

Tell me what happens next?

They might stumble, they might even fall. But then the child gets back up, makes another attempt at it, because they know that one of these days they'll be able to do it. Even the child knows that walking feels a lot better than crawling, and there's no way they're going back to crawling.

Everyone can do it—it doesn't begin with huge giant steps, it starts with small ones. But you must have an open-minded, positive attitude. It's going to be tough, of course. There will definitely be setbacks. You'll have your bad days, but I can also tell you, you'll probably have many more good ones.

Unfortunately, there are no shortcuts. But the sooner you get started, the easier the journey will become. Every step you take, regardless of how small they are, will be "giant" steps in the right direction.

Life is constantly changing, whether you like it or not. When you were young, the only thing that mattered to you was yourself. As you matured, you acquired knowledge and developed friendships and intimate relationships. Then came reality, that new job followed by a promotion, or perhaps a new start-up business. While this was happening maybe you developed a serious relationship, which resulted in marriage. Maybe you decided to have a child, then perhaps another one or two. Then came school, and all the activities that your children were involved in. Before you know it, your personal time becomes less and less. When does your time ever come again? "Probably never!" you might say.

You're right, it could easily be never, if you let it. I talk to so many parents at my martial arts centers, and my usual question to them is, "Why don't you train with us? You know, this is not just for kids...." or "Do you exercise regularly?"

Unfortunately, the answer from most of them is the same. "I have no time between kids and work," "I'm too old for this," or "I'm way too out of shape for exercise."

It's so sad for all of these dedicated parents—for them, their lives are basically over, and the worst thing is that most of them are not even 40 years of age. They think about their childhood and how fun it was. Now all their focus is on their jobs and families—they don't feature in the equation.

Tell me how ridiculous that is! Not even 40 years old and they've already given up. Don't they understand that they, as parents, are the most important thing to their kids?

As parents, we want the very best for our kids. But what happens if we're sick, and even worse, if we are no longer there for them? When are we going to realize that our health is more important than our jobs?

I look at life as a constant juggling act. You have to be able to adapt to the constantly changing equation, but at the same time not forget about yourself. Please exercise regularly!

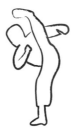

Finding the Fountain of Youth

There are lots of people promoting workout programs that they say will get you in the best shape of your life in a very short amount of time.

Others say that they've developed the perfect diet, where you'll drop a dress size in just a single week. Some claim that you are what you eat, and that juicing is the only way to go. Many say you have to go vegetarian or totally vegan.

And of course, there are those that say, don't even waste your time. There's botox, collagen, cellulite creams, massages, steam and sauna rooms, you name it, we've got it. Just come to our spa for a week and we promise you that you'll feel brand new.

Then there are plastic surgeons that ask why even waste a week when we can make you brand new in a few hours? Just lie back and relax, we'll remove that unwanted fat from anywhere in your body. Want a bigger chest or breasts? Why not let us take care of your abs and butt at the same time with some implants. We'll have you looking great and out in a jiffy.

Maybe I went a bit overboard with the above comparisons, but all these things do happen, every day. Turn on your television set and watch some of the talk shows or infomercials. On one recent show, they were interviewing a doctor while he was performing a live liposuction, and the crazy thing was that the patient wasn't even overweight!

A few months back, a middle-aged couple that I know decided to purchase one of those short-term, quick-fix programs. After doing one session, they told me they were aching for a week, and they had to have massages just to relieve some of the soreness; they never tried doing the program again.

My philosophy has always been if it makes you happy, then it's no one else's business. But one important thing I've learned in my 40-plus years in the fitness industry, is that there's no quick fix when it comes to taking care of one's health and fitness. It should be something that we're concerned about on a daily basis, just like eating and sleeping. If you didn't have a meal, aren't you constantly thinking about food? If you didn't get a good night's sleep, don't you feel groggy throughout the day? Do you ever lose your cool or get stressed out easily? I can tell you that's definitely because you don't exercise regularly.

Sure, it would be great if we were born into a super rich family, or had the looks and body of a supermodel. I don't know how many of you are that lucky, but I for one can tell you that I wasn't that fortunate. Everything I have in my life I owe to the confidence I achieved through Taekwondo. I had to work for everything. Do you think people who are born into wealthy families, or are just naturally beautiful, really appreciate what they have? If you said "yes," why is it that we hear stories all the time about the rich or famous going in and out of rehab, or committing suicide, or going from one relationship one day to another the next?

What would you appreciate more: becoming wealthy by winning the lottery or making a lot of money through your own efforts? You might have said getting lucky winning the lottery, but let's be real. We were not all born with silver spoons in our mouths and the chances of us winning the big jackpot is one in billions. And how many times do you hear stories about lottery winners only ending up even worse off than before they won? Most of these people even say they wish they'd never won the money in the first place. But if you worked really hard to make millions, wouldn't you appreciate it more?

One thing I've learned in life is that nothing is impossible if you're determined enough. I believe that you're in charge of your life and destiny. If you don't take the necessary actions to make things happen, it's not going to happen. I never look at the final destination or my ultimate goal as my driving force. I emphasize each day as my objective. Each and every day should be a goal, where we're learning something about our lives, our jobs, our families and, yes, about our potential.

The problem with most of us is that we don't want to deal with the journey, but just want to get to our destination. It's easy for the aspiring football player to dream about winning the Superbowl in a packed stadium, but few aspiring athletes dream about the endless hours they have to spend training or all the injuries they'll incur. Even if you know someone who has lost a drastic amount of weight, it's easy to look at the "before" and "after" pictures and dream about achieving the same results—but often we don't think about all the hard work and discipline that went into losing that weight. Most of us don't realize it's the journey that teaches us about ourselves. It's the journey that's constantly making us evolve into being a better, healthier, more positive individual.

Happiness is within you, you have to be happy with yourself first. This is easier said than done. How do you go about doing that?

First, you have to take care of yourself by exercising and eating right. Then you have to sit down and think about the good qualities you possess (believe me, you have many). Then you need to look at those qualities you lack or need to improve upon, and work on them.

You might think that's impossible, but I can tell you that you're wrong. Every day in my studio I teach children as young as 3 and as old as 60 or 70. The key thing to remember is to always be open-minded, have the right attitude, be a little humble, and don't think that you know everything, and you'll continue to evolve as an individual.

I've been running my business since I was 22 years old. I've been asked on numerous occasions, especially in an industry where it's so common to open, then close in a short amount of time, or where most instructors teach part-time, "What's the reason for the success of your business?"

I tell everyone that I always strive to give the best in service, best quality of instruction, and make each class fun and goal-oriented. But more importantly, I've learned to adapt to the changing times. That means to be open-minded, not like many grandmasters before me, or the few that are still in the industry, who feel the old way is the only way.

Believe me, there are some things from the old ways I still truly value, such as respect for others and the simplicity of living. But not when it comes to fitness. You mean to tell me the athletes of the past are better than the ones of today? Athletes today are far superior, due to the nutritional knowledge that exists and the better scientific approach that we've developed in training them.

I teach people from all walks of life—students, teachers, police officers, lawyers, stockbrokers, millionaires, celebrities and, yes, even tiny little ones that can barely speak. Some of my older students are more educated than I am, and many are a lot wealthier as well.

So why are they here, what can I offer them? Guess what, that doesn't matter to these individuals. They're here not to compare or compete with one another, but to learn to be the best that they can be. They know that success in life, whether it's a job, relationship, or health, is something that requires constant effort. They know that through exercising they can keep a much clearer head, improve their focus, and not take stress back into their homes. They know that their journey does not end when they get that black belt, or for that matter, a college diploma, a new job, a great test score, or that new relationship, but that they have to be constantly working to be their best, that their efforts are great but they can always do better—to be that best student, worker, lover, or even CEO.

Think how hard one must train to be a champion. But do you know what separates a champion from a great champion and how some of them hold that position until they decide to retire? A great champion does not consider being a champion to be the end of the road, but always thinks that he or she can be even better.

Sometimes I envy my students. They come to take my classes and they have an instructor who can motivate them to work out every day. I wish I had that. I suffered a bad neck and back injury 20 years ago that still bothers me today. At one point, I couldn't even drive because I couldn't turn my neck, so I had to have one of my staff instructors drive me everywhere. Imagine waking up with a stiff neck and not being able to turn your neck. That's what I live with every day.

Add in a knee injury from skiing that was so bad, I couldn't bend my knee for two years. During that time, I used to teach class with my injured leg elevated on a chair! I know I can't train with the same strength and intensity I used to before my injuries, but one thing that got stronger as a result of the injuries is my mind. To continue working out with all those injuries require so much determination and mental strength.

I also believe if I didn't exercise, my injuries would feel even worse than they usually do. Strength and cardio training and stretching go a long way to keeping my body together.

For those with injuries, don't use them as excuses to not exercise, think of them as opportunities to become mentally stronger. If you can apply that same determination you have when exercising to your personal or work life, there's nothing you won't be able to accomplish.

My workouts keep my heart healthy and my body and mind strong. I've found, over the years, that stretching is the biggest factor in looking and feeling young. I can still move and kick like I did 20 or 30 years ago because I stretch. You might be thinking, he's been doing martial arts all his life, he must be naturally flexible. But that isn't the case.

My older brothers were naturally gifted athletes. My oldest brother was not only super flexible, but he had incredible jumping ability. He could easily jump five feet in the air from a standing position. My second-oldest brother had rubberband legs. He could fall asleep in a full side split. He could do a side split on a stack of phone books and his body would dip beyond 180 degrees. He didn't even have to warm up or stretch to do this. Me, I was overweight until I was 13 years old. I couldn't jump and couldn't easily go into a side split like my brothers. I never had the natural ability they had. That's what made me the person I am today. I had to work so much harder than they did to get where I am now.

Former students of mine occasionally come to visit. Students from 10, 15, even 20 years ago! They all tell me the same thing: "Wow! Grandmaster, you look even younger than before!" When they ask how I do it, I tell them working out, eating right, and most importantly, stretching exercises are the path to the fountain of youth.

Teaching Taekwondo is what I do for a living, but that's not what this book is about. I don't expect you to read this book and join your neighborhood Taekwondo studio. But I do want to share with you the workout routines that keep me flexible, strong, and feeling young.

DEVELOPING CONFIDENCE WITH
THE RIGHT ATTITUDE

Most people live without ever understanding what confidence really is. They might have money, looks, a great personality, but still don't have confidence. Sometimes they might be conceited, which can be mistaken for confidence.

Most people are so busy pursuing success that they forget about themselves and ignore their health. Maybe money can make relationships better, but I'm sure you've also heard enough stories about the super rich divorces, where money had just the opposite effect. Also, how can you be sure your partner isn't with you only for your money? Wouldn't you rather they be with you for you and not for your possessions? Which thought makes you feel more confident?

Some people believe confidence is gained through money or looks. I can tell you I'm not one of these people who was born into wealth or is naturally good looking. As a youngster, I was chubby! Confidence was something I had to cultivate.

So what is confidence?

Confidence is believing in yourself and in your convictions, even if that means taking the lonely journey when no one is by your side. It's knowing when to lead by creating your own path, but also understanding that following is okay, too.

Confidence is not being afraid to take risks and knowing that even if what you attempt isn't successful, still you improve by being able to learn from your failures and having the ability to persevere through any setback.

Confidence is knowing when to admit defeat and understanding that failure is a learning process, not the end of the road. It's also being able to bounce back from setbacks when things don't go as planned.

Confidence is understanding that you don't have to be the best, just be the best that you can be. It's being humble enough to praise others and not getting jealous when others succeed. It's being selfless enough to create an easier path for others, especially future generations.

Confidence is knowing you don't need chiseled muscles or six pack abs to look good. It's about being secure enough in yourself to not always be the center of attention. You don't need to make a grand entrance at a party or be the last one to arrive.

Confidence is keeping an open mind and being able to adapt to changes. It's understanding the element of fear by taking precautionary measures. It's knowing that fear is not always your enemy, but can also be your ally.

I believe confidence can be achieved by anyone who's willing to be patient and make an effort. It's attainable through mental and physical conditioning. When I say "patience," I really put emphasis on that word, because this is one quality that most people often overlook or lack.

It is very important to understand that confidence doesn't happen overnight—it's a long and often tedious process that occurs gradually, just like losing weight or getting in shape. One of the rules I've developed through years of teaching is to encourage individuals to set small, short-term goals. My belief is that through small accomplishments, bigger ones become possible; with each new milestone, you will go through changes many times without even realizing them.

To progress, start by making every day a new day. But don't forget yesterday because tomorrow might depend on it. Was yesterday good or bad? If it was good, try to think what made it good and work on those elements that you think made it so good. But if yesterday was bad, think about what went wrong and try your best so that it doesn't happen again. Remember to learn from your mistakes. Too often, we let the same things happen again and again and regret it later. Unless it's the rare thing that you have absolutely no power over, it's your life and you have the ability to control it. Don't make excuses, they will only hurt you more later.

That's why I think martial arts training is so excellent in this matter, because even though most students' long-term goal is to become a black belt, there exists an immediate short-term goal of just trying to achieve the next color belt level (i.e., yellow, green, blue, brown, or red). In order to achieve the next belt level, students must take a performance exam in front of their peers, where with each elevation in rank they are challenged by more difficult testing. What happens is that without even realizing it, these small steps are making their long journey seem shorter and more exciting, since there's something to look forward to at each level. These short-term objectives develop the students into much more confident individuals. And with each elevation in rank, they will be challenged with more difficult skills to learn and be able to execute on the next belt test. With each test, confidence increases little by little.

It's the same with stretching and strengthening. If at first you bend down and your hands can only reach your knees, make it a goal to stretch regularly; so in a week, or two weeks, or a month, your hands can reach your shins. Or if you can only do push-ups from your knees, keep working at it until you can do them balanced on your toes. And keep building on each of your small accomplishments. Think about the things you want in life. You can have these things by developing confidence. I can help you find the way to a life of confidence.

Is there a way to determine if you're becoming a more confident person?

Yes, I believe if you can follow the five tenets of Taekwondo, you're on your way!

CHAPTER 4

Developing Confidence through the Tenets of Taekwondo

Let me give you a brief history of how the five tenets came to be.

In ancient Korea, when it was divided into three kingdoms, a group of fighters were assembled in the Kingdom of Silla, the smallest of the kingdoms. The purpose of this group was to train warriors to defend against the bigger kingdoms. This group was known as the Hwarang and to be considered for selection, a candidate had to have good character and virtue. These candidates were taught art, literature, science and, of course, the art of warfare and hand-to-hand combat. Two of these Hwarang warriors, Kwi-San and Chu-Hang, were responsible for the development of the Hwarang Code of Conduct, which would later evolve into the tenets of Taekwondo. These codes of conduct were:

- Rigid loyalty to king and country
- Respect and obedience to one's parents
- Unwavering loyalty to and trust of friends
- To display courage and never retreat in battle
- Prudence in the use of violence or in the taking of a life

It is this spirit of the Hwarang Code of Conduct that was the root of Silla's morality and strength. And it was through this morality and strength that Silla defeated the two bigger kingdoms—Baekje and Goguryo—which unified the three kingdoms. Out of these codes of conduct, the five tenets of Taekwondo came to be.

- **Courtesy**
- **Integrity**
- **Self-control**
- **Perseverance**
- **Indomitable spirit**

Taekwondo is not just a martial art, it's a way of life—and that's because of these five tenets.

Courtesy

Let's talk about courtesy. It's not just about having good manners and being polite. It's also about respect. Everybody wants respect, I mean, who wouldn't? Think about how good you'd feel if everyone you interacted with treated you with respect? It would be heaven on earth. The thing with respect is if you want it, you have to be willing to give it. When my students bow to me at the Taekwondo school, I'm not just standing there saying, "Yes, bow and worship me!" I'm bowing right back.

It all starts with you. You can change your life by showing respect. Think about going to a job interview. If you greet your interviewer warmly, shake hands using both your hands and address him or her as "sir" or "madam," when it comes to deciding who gets the job, the interviewer will remember how respectful you were, and that can make all the difference.

Or think about a situation you were in where you became angry. Maybe someone cut you off while you were driving or someone bumped into you roughly in the street. In these examples, it becomes a challenge to respond in a courteous manner. The easiest and most instinctive response might be to curse or give the middle finger. Why not try saying, "My mistake, have a great day!" Maybe that person had a really bad day and was just waiting for you to respond in an aggressive manner so they had an excuse to bash you in the head. They might still curse you, but it takes a confident person to let that just roll off their back. The insecure person will most likely retaliate with curses of their own. Nothing diffuses a situation faster than being courteous. If you want to be treated with courtesy, go out of your way to show everyone you are respectful. You'll be known as the person who makes people feel good. That's not a bad reputation to have.

Courtesy doesn't always have to be between people, it can be between you and your environment. I work in New York City and I hear complaints all the time about how dirty the city can be. I was in the subway not too long ago and if you ever rode the New York City subway, you know it's sometimes not the cleanest place in the world. There was a bottle rolling around the floor of the train and of course, whenever it rolled toward someone, they just lifted their feet and let it pass. When it was my stop, as I left, I picked up the bottle and disposed of it. Everyone on the train looked at me like I was crazy, wondering why I would make the effort to clean up someone else's mess. I did it because I wanted the train to look cleaner. If that inspired someone else on the train to do the same, then great. If not, that's okay, too. It's like Ghandi said: "Be the change you want to see in the world."

Integrity

Integrity, in a general sense, means knowing the difference between right and wrong and attempting to do what's right. It means living with honesty. Now of course, this is highly subjective and what's right and wrong may not be the same to everyone. Living with integrity means being true to your family, your friends, the people closest to you. But most importantly, this applies to yourself. I've been in this business over 40 years and part of the reason why I think I've lasted that long is because in all my business transactions, I've always placed a high emphasis on integrity.

Doing the right thing can sometimes be easy, especially if everyone is on board with you. But what about when people disagree with you? Without confidence, you won't be able to stand up for what you believe in or do the right thing. Confidence is living with integrity, even when doing so may cause you to become unpopular or alone.

Self-Control

Self-control also ties in with courtesy and integrity. What I teach my students is a method of attacking and defending that, if not controlled properly, can lead to serious harm or even death. There is a very thin line between defending yourself and becoming the assailant. It's through self-control and integrity that a martial artist is enabled to not cross that line.

The confident person will be able to walk away from a fight because that person knows they have nothing to prove.

Self-control extends beyond just physical altercations. It's the ability to control your emotions and impulses, it's the ability to remain disciplined. Some days, you're not going to want to exercise. Everyone has those days. With all my injuries, even I have those days. Usually, of course, when you feel like that, those are the times that exercising would help the most! You need to be able to control those urges to just sit on the couch and watch TV. I can tell you, I've never felt worse after exercising.

Think about a time when a friend or family member did something to anger you. It's easy to respond with rage, but as you may have experienced, nothing good can come out of that. Remember the first tenet, courtesy? Next time you're in a situation where you feel like responding with anger, use courtesy to control your emotions.

Self-control is involved in something we all do on a daily basis: eating! Sometimes it seems the hardest thing to control is our appetite. It can be a real challenge not to have that extra slice of cake or one more glass of beer. If you want to reach your fitness goals, you have to be able to say no to certain things. We can say "no" to the things we know won't benefit us through the other two tenets—perseverance and indomitable spirit.

Perseverance

Perseverance is dedication. It's following an endeavor no matter the opposition or hardship. Think about where you are in your life now. Would you be there if you didn't have to struggle at some point?

The things that we really appreciate in life are things that we had to work hard to get. You hear stories all the time about people who lost weight. I can promise you they didn't get there by constantly having junk food. It won't be easy and there are times when you'll let temptation beat you. Understand that that's okay. It's okay to fail sometimes. Failure lies not in falling down but in not getting back up.

If one day you go a little overboard with dessert or skip a workout, make a promise to yourself that you won't do that again next time. No matter how hard things get, you have to persist, you have to constantly keep going forward. Whether it's curbing your diet or finding the motivation to exercise, you have to keep at it. Eventually it will become a habit. Did Michael Jordan have a great game every time he played? No. He's had some lousy games. But those are the games that motivated him to work even harder in practice.

I have my students practicing the same blocks and kicks over and over. By the time they become black belts, they must have gone over those techniques thousands of times! Do you think every time they come to a class, they feel like their techniques are improving? No! I can tell you from experience, some days I struggle through my workouts, and my punches and kicks feel incredibly weak. But other days, my body just flows so smoothly, I feel like I can pulverize the punching bag. The only reason I have days like that is through perseverance.

Indomitable Spirit

You can think of perseverance as the physical effort needed to get through a challenge or reach a goal. Indomitable spirit is the intangible inner strength needed to achieve that goal. It's the will to go on regardless of the outcome. Whether you're trying to push through that last rep or run that final mile, it's not giving up, no matter how tired or far behind you are. I try to exercise every day. Do I feel one hundred percent every time I work out? No. But no matter how tired I am or how lousy I feel, I push myself to finish that workout.

Indomitable spirit teaches us that it's the process, not the outcome, that makes us stronger.

Again, like all the previous tenets, this applies not just to exercising. If you've ever lost someone or something close to you, you already understand the role indomitable spirit plays in helping you through those moments of pain and sadness. Indomitable spirit comes in many forms.

It could be your belief in yourself or the memory of a loved one, or through religion. No matter where you draw your inner strength from, giving it your all, even when the odds are stacked against you, is what indomitable spirit is all about.

The ultimate goal of following these five tenets is to achieve our goals and better ourselves. Just to be clear: these tenets are not a religion. They were based on Buddhist principles but the principles found in the tenets are not limited just to Buddhism, or even Eastern philosophy. They can be followed by anyone, from any religion or ideology. In fact, they are compatible with many of the world's major religions. The ideals of courtesy and respect, loyalty and integrity, perseverance and courage are all found throughout religious texts and teachings.

Right now, as you read this, there are wars going on all over the world because of differences in religion and ideology. Can you imagine how peaceful the world would be if everyone genuinely adopted these tenets? Trying to end war and conflict is ambitious to say the least. It's a lot to take on and a lot of it is out of our control, but what we can control is conflict in our personal lives and our relationships with other people. One step at a time. That's what this book is about.

A MESSAGE FOR PARENTS

One thing I've learned through the years of teaching children is that parents sometimes enroll their kids in too many different activities and sports, thinking because they're doing so many different things, this will help them develop confidence faster. But I believe what usually ends up happening is the opposite. This is especially true for team sports. Don't get me wrong, I believe team sports can be a great way for kids to learn camaraderie and the importance of teamwork, but not so much for developing confidence, unless your child is the star player on the team.

If your child is not great in their sport, they won't get a lot of opportunities to play; instead, he or she's usually on the sideline—which is not great for confidence. Even professional athletes lose confidence and doubt their abilities when their coach benches them for another player. Even if it's a pick-up game amongst friends, what usually happens is that the best players are assigned captains and they pick who they want on their team. This may have happened to you as a youngster. If you're one of the first kids picked for teams, that's great; but what about the child that's begrudgingly picked last?

The other issue with not just team sports, but competitive sports, is the idea of competition. Yes, competition can make you better or make you work harder, but if your only focus in life is to try to be better than someone else, your goal will always be dependent on the actions of others. If your competitor decides to take it down a notch, do you do that as well? Or if your competitor's giving it one hundred percent, do you only then give one hundred percent? Also, you will always be comparing yourself to others, which is not the best for developing confidence.

Competitive sports can be a great way to test your skills against your peers and it can be extremely rewarding, so if a student approaches me and asks for help in preparing for a tournament, I won't brush them off. But as I said, if that's your only focus, it can be very limiting in terms of developing happiness and confidence. I know what you're thinking: look at this martial arts guy talking about competition—isn't that all they do, beat up on each other like on TV or in the movies? Unfortunately, from a certain perspective I can see why people think that way. But the truth is that in "real" martial arts we seek to train students to be the best they can be. It's more about building confidence and living a healthier lifestyle than fighting.

I know there are many martial arts centers out there that only train for competition. If that's your preference, that's up to you. But I can tell you there are many more that teach individuals not just about fighting, but about the philosophy to be a more honest, healthy, and humble person—because the real truth is that a person who possesses these qualities is much more confident.

When I was in my twenties, I competed in many martial arts tournaments. I won't lie and say I won all of them. I lost a lot more than I won, but whether I lost or won, I always made it a goal to give one hundred percent every time. So even when I lost a sparring match, I still walked away with confidence. Over time, I realized being a competitor can be extremely selfish, because when you're training to become a champion, you are only concerned about one person—yourself! I decided to take a different approach and realized that instead of just seeking to make myself a champion, I could make multiple champions—not just in tournaments, but also in life, which is much more satisfying. I understand that as parents, we want to give our children the opportunities that we might not have had growing up, but please try not to overburden your children with too many activities. If possible, enroll your child in at least one activity that places an emphasis on individual achievement and overall mental and physical well-being. Think "quality over quantity."

That's not to say if your child is a prodigy at a team sport like baseball to take him or her out of little league. If an activity is contributing to your child becoming more confident, then by all means, keep him or her involved.

Maybe this will be biased, but I highly recommend enrolling your child in martial arts. Not only will your child get stronger and fitter, but he or she will develop focus, concentration and confidence. Unless you are involved with martial arts, it is also one of the few activities with which you won't be able to help your child. Knowing their parents can't help them remember a form or learn a new kick instills a sense of personal responsibility and achievement within children.

With bullying becoming a huge issue, your child will also have a better chance of defending themself if the situation arises. Unfortunately, bullies tend to go after people who look like they can't stand up for themselves. If children know that they can defend themselves when push comes to shove, their confidence can be seen through their body language.

Michael Imperioli's Thoughts on the Tenets of Taekwondo

Through practicing the tenets of Taekwondo, I've become a more patient, calmer, and confident person. I know I've become a healthier person.

I've found that courtesy is taken for granted and not considered to be very important. They say you'll catch more flies with honey. If you're kind, things go easier in life in general. Living in New York, everyone is rushing all the time. If you take a minute to say "hello," or smile at someone, or say "thank you," or give up a seat on the subway, if you make that a real point in your life to be present enough to be kind and generous and considerate and respectful, your world will become better. People respond to those things and they'll give it back. The more you do that, the more you're going to see that in your world. We're all connected, we all live on the same planet, and the more you practice tenets like that, the more you're going to see it in the world and the happier you're going to be.

I find that as an actor, my concentration levels have increased dramatically since I started martial arts. Over the years I've done a lot of fight scenes and martial arts just made it a lot easier to stay healthy doing that stuff because you're repeating the same moves over and over and doing so many takes. And doing martial arts allowed me to do stuff like that without getting injured and helped my control during fight scenes.

In acting, you need concentration and relaxation. Martial arts has definitely helped my concentration level. I find it easier to learn lines now. I think by exercising and practicing martial arts and committing to that kind of mental focus on a regular basis, it's helped my work. It's helped me stay in the moment more. Because when you're acting and the cameras are rolling, you need to be in the moment and block everything else out. Martial arts are very conducive to this type of work.

People have all kinds of perceptions about martial arts. The first thing most people will ask when they find out you do martial arts is, "Did you ever have to use it?" I haven't had to use it in a confrontational situation, but it becomes a part of who you are, it becomes your instinct. It's funny because in the years before I started, there were a couple of physical confrontations that I got into, and it was probably because I wasn't practicing martial arts that I got into them. At the time, my vibe was tuned into a more aggressive level; whereas after practicing martial arts for a long period of time, you start to go beyond that. And you're not giving off that aggression or fear.

Over time, friends and family who know I do Taekwondo have seen the results and have seen me become a calmer and more thoughtful person. They really admire it. They don't quite know what it is we do—they think it's about fighting and learning how to break somebody's arm. I mean, that's definitely there and you will learn how to defend yourself, but there's so much more. I don't know everything about all the martial arts disciplines, but I'm sure they all have their benefits. I tell people it's always about the teacher. Grandmaster Kang somehow instills in you not only the desire to push yourself, but also the confidence that you can push yourself past what you thought were your limits.

And he does it in a way that he feels almost more like a friend than a teacher. He is a teacher but you also feel like he's a friend who cares about you. If your family's there, he cares about your children too. The children's program here is very successful and I think it's because people trust their children to be in this environment because of what he instills. He really lives these tenets. He's one of the kindest, most courteous, respectful, and thoughtful people I've ever met.

I took a karate class for a couple of months about 20 years ago, to prepare for a film where I played a martial arts instructor. And the Grandmaster of this school was really overweight. I never saw him work out. I don't know if he did. Once in a while, he'd show up and give a little speech, but that was it.

You have to be an example. If you really want to tell your kids to do something, you have to practice what you preach first. If I'm following an unhealthy diet, it's hard to tell my kids not to do the same.

Here, you have a teacher who's running a school who's in tremendous physical shape, who is still perfecting the art of Taekwondo. When you watch him train, you really see the beauty of the art. And I've never heard him yell or seen him enraged. I've seen him deal with difficulty from time to time. I've spent a lot of time with him and I've never seen him lose his cool, ever. He teaches by example—what it is to be a good human being, and a happy and a healthy human being, and really practice what you preach.

CHAPTER 5

Exercise and Food Plan for Life

There are countless ways to exercise but to simplify things, I'll break them into three categories: you have strength training, usually done by lifting weights; cardio training, usually done through running, cycling, or swimming; and you have stretching, usually in the form of yoga. Each of these are great ways to work out. But I think they would be even more beneficial as a supplement to my form of training.

For many of us, we need to exercise not just to stay healthy but also to relieve stress. With the United States barely out of the great recession, if you currently have a job, hanging on to that job is stressful. And if you're looking for a job, there's not a lot of opportunity out there, so that's also a big contributor to stress. We need ways to release all this stress now more than ever. Strength training and yoga are good ways to stay active, but don't have the same tension release that you get from a martial arts style workout. With strength training and yoga, the emphasis is on strengthening the body by bringing energy into the body. Whether you're pulling a weight or holding a pose in yoga, you're channeling all that energy and tension back into the body.

Cardio training is also a good form of exercise. But you have to be very careful. Some of you reading this may have knee or hip problems from years of running. So many of my students who ran in their twenties and thirties are now suffering because of all those years of impact on their knees and hips. Even my students who used to get their cardio exercise through cycling tell me they have back pain from being hunched over on their bikes.

Have you ever been so stressed that you screamed your lungs out or cried your eyes out? How did you feel afterward? I'm willing to bet you felt like a great weight had been lifted off your body. When you're stressed, you need that release. My method of exercise combines strength training, cardio, and stretching. The method of stretching I use is different from the method used in yoga. Instead of holding a position like in yoga, you're moving and using the dynamic stretches in Taekwondo. My system of stretching is meant to not only release tension from the body—it will also keep your joints loose and body flexible. I place a great deal of emphasis on stretching the legs. Our legs contain some of the biggest muscles in our body and because of this, not only do we burn more calories by utilizing these muscles, but our blood circulation also improves.

As we get older, our mobility and flexibility decreases. By stretching, not only do we keep our body flexible—which makes us feel more youthful—but we also prevent a lot of common injuries.

One of the main aspects of Taekwondo training is "Forms" training. You can think of a form as being similar to what boxers do when they shadow box, except in Taekwondo, it's a set of movements you have to memorize. These movements consists of stances, blocks, and strikes, using the hands and feet. Balance, strength, cardio, and concentration are all involved. It's also a form of meditation. If you've trained in a martial art that involves forms, you may know them by the terms *Hyung*, *Poomse*, or *Kata*.

When you're at the gym or out running, there are so many distractions. You have music, TV, people on their phones, people talking to you; but when you're doing these forms, you have to be able to block out all distractions. If you're thinking about work or what's for dinner while you do these forms, you will lose your place. This is why I, and other practitioners of Taekwondo, feel so much better after a workout. For the duration of the workout, you're blocking all your worries and stress out of your head. Even if it's for just 30 minutes, that 30 minutes can carry on into the rest of your day. That "mental workout" of blocking the outside world while we're training is just as important as the physical workout.

Strengthening Plan Outline

When anyone mentions weight training, it seems like a no-brainer. Nowadays everyone seems to know that having a lean, solid physique not only looks great, but also combats some of the conditions that are associated with aging, like osteoporosis (loss of bone density), sarcopenia (loss of muscle mass), or arthritis.

Also, we've learned that increasing muscle mass will develop greater coordination and balance, help avoid the loss of joint flexibility, and assist in preventing injuries. And now, more recent studies are showing even greater benefits of strength training, such as reducing the risk of diabetes. Because developing muscle tissue increases the number of proteins that help pull glucose/sugar from the bloodstream and use it for energy, this in turn will help lower overall blood sugar levels.

When it comes to developing muscles, women always tell me the same thing: "If I lift too much I'm going to get bulky, I don't want that." My answer to them is always the same: since men have increased levels of testosterone, they will increase in muscle size, but for women, strength training will tone you rather than give you huge muscles, so don't worry.

It's also common for men to ask what kind of development they'll get using light weights. Recent studies show that doing high reps with light weights can produce greater strength gains than previously thought.

Another thing I always stress to people is that I'm talking about strength training, not bodybuilding. Bodybuilders are in a whole different category. These individuals have a level of discipline and commitment like no other. I'm not saying my strength training regimen is at the opposite end of the scale, but it's nowhere as intense, so you don't have to make such demands on yourself. My philosophy of exercise aims for overall health and well-being for the rest of your life.

My strength training program is a bit different: first of all, the rep count is not as important as the time spent on each exercise.

Secondly, I don't want you to rest in-between exercises—this way you'll keep your heart rate up.

Third, I want you to use light weights, where there is less chance of injury. I encourage you to do as many reps as possible within a specified time.

Finally, I emphasize the frequency of doing these strength training exercises three times per week. Yes, repeat the whole sequence three times a week. I'm sure all of you are used to hearing about working each body part once a week, but I want you to do these exercises three times per week.

Look at the philosophy behind physical therapy. If you've ever gotten injured and had to do physical therapy, you had to build the muscle back up every day, not just once a week. And instead of lifting heavy weights, you use light weights with high reps.

I have nothing against lifting heavy weights. I used to lift heavy weights too, and I enjoyed it. But I also sustained many injuries that way.

Heavy weights are good when you're young, but if you're older and get injured, at best, you can't work that body part for a while. At worst, you might not be able to work out at all until you recover. Why put your body at so much risk when lifting light weights can give you the same, if not better, results as lifting really heavy weights?

For over three decades, back when almost all of the weightlifters at the gym were lifting heavy weights, I've primarily trained with light weights. Besides not wanting to take the chance of injuring myself and missing competitions, I found light weights not only made me stronger, but also improved my martial arts skills and overall fitness. If I had huge muscles like a giant body builder, there's no way I could move the way I do.

I group my exercises into weekly increments, where the first two weeks concentrate on simple calisthenic routines (using just your body weight), emphasizing the three major parts of the body: upper body, legs, and core.

During the third and fourth weeks, I add dumbbell exercises in addition to the calisthenics, working on shoulders, back, triceps, and biceps. Finally, during the last two weeks and from then on, I introduce leg exercises in conjunction with upper body dumbbell routines for an added cardio training.

This will not only up the cardio factor: it also engages the core, as well as balance and mimicks motions you would use on a daily basis. You might think that to build muscle, you need to isolate the muscle with exercises that target just that specific muscle group, but the way our bodies move, we rarely use just one muscle group at a time. You use muscles in your legs, core, arms, and shoulders just picking something up off the floor.

There's nothing wrong with just doing bicep curls if you want to build more bicep strength or work on definition, but you'll get a greater overall body workout by doing bicep curls with lunges.

When you're working out, don't be afraid to break a sweat. I know that might sound like strange advice, but in my many decades in the fitness industry, I've met many people who worked out only at a slow to moderate pace. When I asked them why, the answer I heard most often was, "I don't like to sweat."

Sweating is good for you! It's your body's way of cooling you when your body temperature rises due to activity. It also helps with losing weight.

It's also incredibly relaxing. If you're stressed and you work up a sweat, you will feel a lot calmer and more relaxed.

COMBINED DYNAMIC STRETCHING

My "Combined Dynamic Stretching" method is a very different way of stretching, because it doesn't just focus on flexibility, but also works on improving balance, cardio, strength, and mental focus as well. Since most of my exercises are combined movements, they'll stretch multiple parts of the body simultaneously, improving circulation, while warming up the body for physical activity and helping prevent injuries.

Starting with upper body stretches, I'll make you hold at the beginning and end points of a specific stretch, then make you repeat the same stretch while gradually increasing the speed and range of the motion. Then, through leg stretches, I'll not only work your muscles, but the core regions of the body, where often the greatest amount of tension lies, engaging in focused core strength training exercises. Finally, I'll take you to the floor, where you'll get a chance to do stretching routines while seated or lying back, instead of standing and putting added strain on the body. Here, the emphasis will be less about balance or cardio and more focused on recovery.

Whether you're a beginner or a veteran to stretching, I've created a seven week, bi-weekly set of routines for you to follow and keep you challenged. In the beginner phase, during the first two weeks, it's all about doing basic fundamental stretches for the entire body, something that I recommend doing daily to get you charged-up. Two weeks later, in the intermediate phase, I start working on your core region and your large leg muscles by incorporating various types of standing stretches, to develop not just linear but also lateral mobility and strength. In the advanced phase it gets even more exciting, because now the bulk of your stretching regimen is based on Taekwondo-type kicking moves. In Taekwondo, flexibility is an integral part of training. We don't do stretching exercises just to feel loose, but more in preparation to execute proper kicks.

Mostly, all my stretching exercises are based on the martial arts concept of forms training, meaning they are routines created not just to help your flexibility, but also to improve your concentration. In your final level, the "black belt phase," I've created a 40-movement "stretching form" that will work your entire body, emphasizing all the important areas of exercise as previously mentioned: balance, strength, cardio, flexibility, and focus. Do this stretching form five times in a row, at different speeds, to help relieve your mind and body of unwanted tension and stress.

The key to improving or developing greater flexibility is not to overdo it, but to build gradually and consistently. Also note that tension is an enemy to stretching, so in order to decrease this, proper breathing is very important. Usually, the rule of breathing is to exhale when you're exerting pressure, which will help your body alleviate the tension and keep you relaxed during the stretching move.

If possible, make stretching a "life's habit," meaning it should be done every day. It is ideal to do some light stretches (foundation stretches) every day when you wake up, or when you feel stiff from sitting too long, or even to help with a job that's physically demanding.

The stretching exercises that I have created are not just for this book, but are exercises that I've been incorporating into my classes for several decades, and something that I do on a daily basis. A true testament to how successful any fitness program is should not be determined simply by the number of participants, but more by how long they stick with it. To date, I have trained over 20,000 people and awarded more than 2,000 students the rank of black belt or higher. The minimum time for anyone to achieve a black belt, regardless of their ability, is 24–30 months. So if all these people are sticking with my training program for that much time, it has to be working for them.

All this is to say that what I teach is not a trend or a new fad. It's a proven method of exercise that will increase your energy and focus and help prevent injuries, either from your daily functions or whatever activities you engage in.

Eating Habits

Most people around the world don't know what three meals a day is. As a matter of fact, most people are happy just having a single meal a day, not by choice of course, but because of shortages or financial circumstance.

I came to this country in 1969 from South Korea, a country that had been occupied by Japan for almost four decades and had then suffered a civil war. I experienced hunger firsthand. It was so common to just have one meal a day. No, it wasn't a huge meal with salad, pasta, steak, and potatoes, followed by dessert. It was more along the lines of a bowl of rice with some simple vegetables. Maybe, if we were lucky, there might have been some eggs or fish. As for meat, we ate it a handful of times during the year, on special occasions.

There are millions of people around the world that still live and work on a daily basis with limited food intake, and they're surviving. What I'm trying to say is that we don't need to eat three meals a day, especially big ones. As a matter of fact, most of us tend to overeat, which decreases our energy throughout the day. It is common practice for Buddhist monks to fast for long periods, sometimes for a week or even longer, while only drinking water. Their belief is that by constantly eating every few hours, your body focuses its energy on digestion and that by fasting you can utilize the energy to strengthen your mind and develop a heightened level of concentration.

I'm sure you have noticed the "super-size" concept, but guess what? That's only really in America. If you travel around the world there is no such thing elsewhere. The worst part is the kids' menu in restaurants. It's crazy—burgers and fries, mac and cheese, chicken fingers, etc. We're feeding junk food to our kids, then, on top of that, we give them ridiculous portions. "But they don't want to eat anything else!" This is a common phrase I hear from parents. Maybe if we don't expose them to all the junk food that's out there, and don't give them so many choices, they'll eat healthier. Do you know what the real problem is? It's us—as grown-ups and parents, we must set the proper example first. In martial arts we have a saying that some of you might have heard before: "It's never a bad student, it's a bad teacher."

When you eat Asian food, there is no such thing as a piece of steak for one person—meat is usually cut into pieces and combined with vegetables or noodles. Obviously this style developed due to the lack of meat, but if you think about it, notice how well-balanced that concept is. Don't get me wrong, I'm not advocating an all-vegetarian or vegan diet, I love a steak or burger as much as the next person. But if you can reduce the amount of meat you consume and add more vegetables, it will help with the weight loss as well as some of the negative effects of eating too much meat, like high blood pressure or heart disease.

We live in age of abundance and comfort, especially in America—huge cars, homes, and mostly a lot of food. Many food experts say we should break up our meals to six per day. More power to the person with that much time on their hands. I don't know about you, but between running my martial arts studios, teaching, exercising, and spending time with my family and friends, I don't have enough hours in the day to eat six meals.

To make it easier, many diet plans will send pre-packaged meals to your doorstep, which is great if you have the money and you're home all day. But, I'm guessing it's not going to be too convenient for the person that works (not from home) or is running around doing chores—or both. Do they expect you to take the meals and a microwave with you wherever you go?

There are differing opinions on how many meals you should eat in a day, whether it should be six or three, or even one big one. The only thing nutritionists can agree on is that the only way to lose weight is to burn more calories than you consume. If the average person burns 2,000 calories without any exercise, just from being alive, then eating less than 2,000 calories is the only way to lose weight (we're not factoring in exercise for this example).

The bottom line is this, if you absolutely have to drop weight quickly (whether it's for medical reasons or just to get you motivated), take the normal portion of food you eat at every meal and eat only half. This will not be easy and will require a lot of discipline, but reducing your food intake by half is more than sufficient for your body.

You might be thinking, "what a crazy diet!"

You're absolutely right, but if you can do it, you'll see amazing results.

But as you can see, an eating regimen like this can only be temporary, possibly for a few days, because even though our bodies won't care, our minds will not let it happen. It cannot be an eating plan for the rest of your life.

3 – 2 – 1 Eating Plan For Life

This is when my "3-2-1 Eating Plan For Life" can help you. It's an eating plan that won't feel like a shock to the body. It's gradual, easy to follow, and best and most important of all, it's something we can do for the rest of our lives. It's not one of those 8 week or 3 month diet programs where you're feeling miserable and craving all your favorite foods.

I'm sure you've seen infomercials late at night advertising some get rich quick schemes. Do you really think they all work, have you ever met someone that had success with any of them? It's the same with these short, intense diet or exercise regimens. Sure, you might get some results within the time frame but what about after? Studies show people who engage in diets not only gain all the weight they lost after coming off the diet, but actually end up gaining even more weight than when they first started. So my method is not a quick fix plan, it is something you can do as long as you like, that's why I really can't call it a "diet."

It's a method of eating whereby we try to re-train our minds and make them think they're still getting what they want. The truth is, in reality it *is* getting what it wants, just in a different sequence. My method is to simply reverse your daily meal portions, by making your breakfast (3) the biggest meal of the day, lunch (2) the second, and your dinner (1) the smallest. If you think about it, normally it's 1-2-3, where breakfast is usually the smallest meal (if you even eat breakfast at all), lunch is the second biggest meal, and dinner is the biggest meal of the day.

I know what works in the long run, not just for myself but for my students as well. When my students come to me for advice on an eating plan, I always tell them to follow this method that I've been doing for decades. Since you are more active during the day, your body will have more time to convert the calories into energy rather than storing them as fat. Dinner should be smaller because your body will not have time to digest before sleep like during the day. It's best that you eat enough during the day so you won't feel the need to overeat at night. You might initially feel like the amount you eat for dinner is not enough, but the food that you ate earlier in the day will be more than enough to carry you through the night. Also try not to snack late at night, this is an easy way to ruin your healthy eating habits.

If you're a morning exercise person, I recommend that you try to do so on an empty stomach (of course water is never considered food). If that's very difficult for you to do, have small snack like a fruit, cereal bar, oatmeal, etc., then after your workout have that large breakfast I was talking about.

Remember that maintaining a regular exercise regimen is the key to weight loss. Exercising is more vital and it should either come first or in conjunction with any eating plan. It will stimulate you and give you the confidence that will help you to make healthier food choices.

Taekwondo Belt System

The way my strengthening, stretching, and eating plans are designed, each week represents a belt level. In my Taekwondo system, we start at white belt, then yellow, green, blue, brown, red, and finally black.

- White represents the innocence and clean slate of a beginner.
- Yellow represents the seed of Taekwondo that has been planted.
- Green represents the color of growth as the seed matures into a plant.
- Blue is for the sky to which the plant aims to reach.
- Brown represents the soil from which the plant continues to sustain its energy.
- Red is the color of blood and fire, so it represents the danger, power, and passion of the practitioner.
- Black represents maturity and the understanding and knowledge of the previous color belt levels.

In Taekwondo, the different color belts denote knowledge of the forms and required skills for that particular belt level. The colors also represent how long someone has been training (the more advanced the belt, the longer that person has been training). Belts also serve as a motivational tool. They make the journey from white belt to black belt more manageable.

This is why the belt system in Taekwondo is so important. When I trained as a child, before the color belt system became implemented, there were only white belts and black belts. Everyone started as a white belt and kept that belt. It only turned black through the many years of sweat and dirt (and occasionally blood) that came from training.

If I told a new white belt that their next belt would be a black belt, which they would receive after two to three years of training, I doubt any of them would stick with the curriculum. But if I told them, after a few months, they would test for their yellow belt, the journey to black belt doesn't seem so arduous.

Too often, after my red belts test for their black belts, they see that as the end of their Taekwondo journey. But, I tell them, it's really the beginning. Now that they have an understanding of the basic techniques they learned through color belts, it's time to put all that knowledge to good use. It's like taking a driver's ed course with the goal of passing the road test just to receive your driver's license! The driver's license represents the skills you've acquired to be a good driver, so why not put it to use?

As important as weight loss and physical health are, your mental strength and attitude also play a key part. For each level, you should try to follow this mindset.

WHITE BELT BEGINNER LEVEL (WEEK ONE)— LET'S KEEP IT SIMPLE

Welcome to your new life! Every trip begins with a single step, and this is it. As a beginner, or white belt, you must have an open-minded approach toward exercise and eating.

Take it easy, start slowly—you don't want to be intimidated by the word "exercise." Like a baby, you're taking your first walking steps. Don't try to run before you can walk.

Let's try to work on building the right foundation—by that, I mean attitude. Positive attitude is what's going to get you going and keep you going. Just like in life, there are always setbacks. Understand it takes time and devotion, don't give up after a day or two.

Especially at this beginning level, don't jump on and off the scale ten times a day or tell yourself that you have to lose 40 pounds within three months. That's like a 10-year-old telling himself he's going to master throwing a curveball in three months. If only it was that easy.

I'm not trying to dissuade you, but don't set long-term goals at this stage. As a beginner, you want to take it day by day, step by step. If you put high expectations on what you need to accomplish at this level, you're going to be putting too much of a burden on yourself and constantly be disappointed. I'm sure we've all heard the saying, you're your own worst enemy.

When someone engages in physical exercise, they're very focused on the end result or their final destination. But what they forget to see is that their goal is not what's going to change them—instead, it's the effort you've made or the drive to get there that has already changed you.

Daily goals or short-term goals are what you need to focus on. Like a child, we have to teach our bodies and minds to do simple tasks—"I think I can handle this," is what you should be saying. Also, when doing most exercise moves, perform them in a moderate manner. You're not trying to perfect these moves overnight. Think of yourself sculpting a bust—you're not going take that chunk of clay and start making the eyes. Create a general foundation. That means focus on getting yourself to move first—it might not look perfect, but it's a start.

It's like training for a marathon. You're not going to try to run 20 miles on the first day of training. You might start off with one mile the first day, then two the next, and so on.

Do you remember how you learned the alphabet? First you sang it as a song, then you learned each letter in detail—A, B, C. It's the same with losing weight.

This stage is the most crucial, because often we don't even give ourselves a chance. We forget that we didn't gain the excess weight overnight, but we feel that we have to lose it immediately. Have some patience!

Strengthening Plan Week 1: White Belt Beginner Level

Strength goals:

1. Condition the larger muscle groups of the body by performing fundamental calisthenic exercises using your body weight.
2. Try to perform each exercise for a minimum of 30–60 seconds, with about the same amount of rest time in-between the exercises.
3. Depending on your personal fitness level, you can always moderate the speed, intensity, or time duration of each exercise, even repeating the whole sequence if possible.
4. Try to perform these exercise three days this first week, skipping a day in-between.

Note: Movement—Perform each exercise in a controlled manner, not too fast or abruptly, avoiding any excessive motion.

Breathing—Always inhale when contracting and hold for a moment, then exhale when moving again.

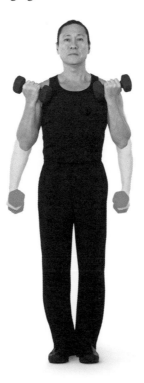

UPPER BODY

1. PUSH-UPS (chest, shoulders, back, arms) 30–60 seconds

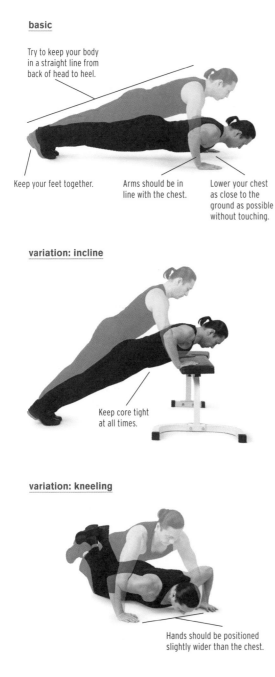

basic

Try to keep your body in a straight line from back of head to heel.

Keep your feet together.

Arms should be in line with the chest.

Lower your chest as close to the ground as possible without touching.

variation: incline

Keep core tight at all times.

variation: kneeling

Hands should be positioned slightly wider than the chest.

Push-ups are the best callisthenic exercise. Even though push-ups are considered a chest exercise, they really work your entire body—top to bottom, including the core region, and can be modified to suit your personal fitness level.

Start Position—Body facing the floor, hands slightly wider than shoulders with palms in line with the chest and facing down on the floor, feet together.

Movement—Keeping the body as straight as possible, bend both arms, lowering your chest as close to the floor as possible without touching, then extend your arms, pushing your body back up—but do not fully extend your arms or "lock" your elbows.

Performance—Hold slightly at the bottom and never lock your arms at the top. Perform for 30–60 seconds.

Breathing—Inhale when lowering the chest.

Variations: kneeling and incline

LOWER BODY

2. LEG SQUATS (quads, hamstrings, glutes, calves) 30–60 seconds

Start Position—Stand upright with feet shoulder width apart.

Movement—Try to lower your body so that the top of your thighs are as close as possible to parallel with the floor, and hold slightly at the lowest point. Keep the body upright; making sure the knees don't go farther forward than the toes when bending. Squeeze tight the glutes and hamstrings on the upward movement, but don't fully lock legs.

Performance— Perform continuously for 30–60 seconds.

Breathing—Inhale at the lowest position.

Variation: chair squat

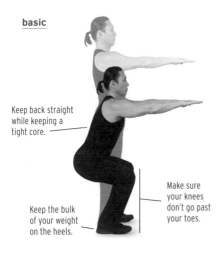

basic

Keep back straight while keeping a tight core.

Keep the bulk of your weight on the heels.

Make sure your knees don't go past your toes.

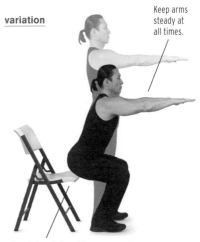

variation

Keep arms steady at all times.

Use chair only to guide you, never to fully support all your body weight.

CORE

3. LYING BACK BENT LEG LIFTS 30–60 seconds

Lying back with knees bent and hands flat on the floor to the sides of the body, lift hips and legs off the floor, pulling the knees to the chest in a rolling motion, then slowly lower your legs without touching the floor.

Variation: two motion straight leg lift—lift hips and legs straight off the floor, then lower body, extending the legs downward without touching the floor.

basic

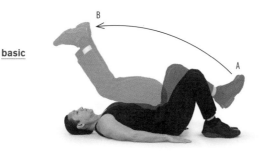

START POSITION–Lie back with knees bent and feet on the floor with arms by your side.

MOVEMENT–With legs bent, pull both knees to your chest picking your hips and legs off the floor, then lower.

PERFORMANCE–Perform in a rolling motion continuously for 30-60 seconds.

BREATHING–Exhale when knees are at the chest.

variation

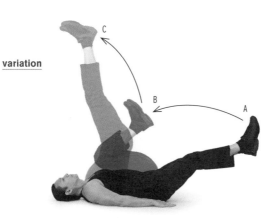

START POSITION–Legs extended off the floor.

MOVEMENT–Bend both knees to your chest, followed by an upward thrust, where your legs hips, and lower back are lifted off the floor. When lowering your legs, reverse the sequence.

PERFORMANCE–30-60 seconds.

BREATHING–Exhale when legs are at highest point.

Stretching Plan Week 1: White Belt Beginner Level

Stretching goals:

1. Understanding the importance of daily stretching by performing standing foundation stretches when first waking up, to help promote greater circulation and fluidity of the body.
2. Perform foundation floor stretches in conjunction with the standing stretches; this can also be done at the end of the day before bed, to help alleviate the tension of a long day.
3. Foundation stretches are very gentle stretches, they can be done throughout the day, either in segments or as a whole, anytime you feel tense.
4. Foundation stretches should be done at least three days minimum this week.

Note: Movement—Perform each exercise in a gradual and constant manner, while trying to reach or extend farther with each repetition.

Breathing—Always exhale while exerting pressure.

Just like washing your face or brushing your teeth, these exercises should be a daily life habit. They can also be performed as warm up or cool down exercises for the strengthening exercises.

STANDING FOUNDATION STRETCHES

1. NECK STRETCHES

   Start Position—Stand up straight with feet shoulder width apart and arms by your side.

   Breathing—Breathe normally and maintain a relaxed facial expression.

   A. NECK LIFTS—Tilt head down (hold), then tilt up (hold), then up and down, four times.
   B. NECK TILTS—Lower the ear to right shoulder (hold), then left (hold), then back and forth, four times.
   C. NECK TURNS—Turn head to right (hold), then left (hold), then back and forth, four times.
   D. NECK ROTATIONS—Drop the head and rotate fully to the right, then to the left, four times.

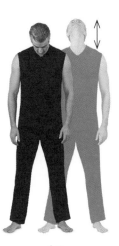

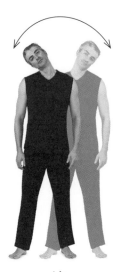

MOVEMENT–Slowly tilt the head down, holding at the lowest position for two seconds, then tilt the head up and hold for two seconds. Only hold the position the first time. Gently go through the entire range of motion, tilting your head down then up at a normal pace.

PERFORMANCE–Repeat the up and down movements for four reps.

MOVEMENT–Slowly tilt your head sideways as if you were trying to touch your ear to your shoulder.

Hold your head at the lowest point for two seconds, then repeat on the other side.

PERFORMANCE–Only hold once at each position in the beginning.

1.a

1.b

Your forehead-to-chin axis should be vertical.

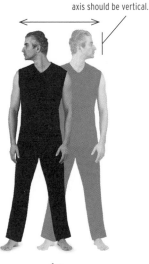

MOVEMENT–Slowly turn your head to the side as far as you can go, holding at the farthest point for two seconds, then repeat on the other side. Make sure not to turn your body in the direction of the head turn.

PERFORMANCE–Repeat the side-to-side turning motion for a total of four times at a normal pace. Only hold once at each turning position in the beginning.

MOVEMENT–Start in a head-down position. Gently rotate the neck in a circular motion, completing a full circle in one direction, then repeat in the other direction. It should take a minimum of five seconds to complete one full rotation. Inhale while rotating the head upward and exhale while rotating down.

PERFORMANCE–Complete four full neck rotations two times in each direction, alternating from one direction to the other.

1.c

1.d

2. SHOULDER STRETCHES

Start Position—Stand upright with feet shoulder width apart and arms by your sides.

Breathing—Breathe normally.

A. UP/DOWN SHRUGS—Shrug both shoulders up (hold), and down (hold), then up and down, four times.

B. FRONT/BACK SHRUGS— Bring both shoulders forward (hold), and back (hold), then back and forth, four times.

C. SHOULDER ROTATIONS— Rotate both shoulders forward four times and backward four times.

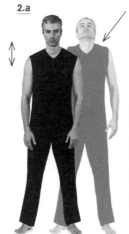

2.a

Hold and squeeze at the highest point for two seconds.

MOVEMENT—Lift both shoulders as high as possible holding at the top and then gently lowering them.

Only hold and squeeze the first time.

PERFORMANCE—Repeat for a total of eight reps.

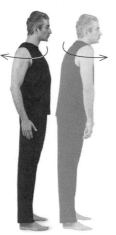

MOVEMENT—Bring both shoulders inward to the chest, rounding off your upper back area, then squeeze and hold for two seconds. Bring both shoulders back as if squeezing them together and then hold for two seconds (chest area should be rounded off).

PERFORMANCE—Bring both shoulders in and then back, performing in a continuous manner for four reps. Only hold once in the beginning of the exercise.

2.b

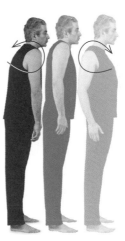

MOVEMENT—Gently roll both shoulders backward in a smooth, circular manner, then roll them forward.

PERFORMANCE—Perform in a continuous circular manner, four times in one direction, then four times in the opposite direction.

2.c

3. ARM STRETCHES

Start Position—Stand upright with feet shoulder width apart and arms by your sides.

Breathing—Breathe normally.

A. FRONT/BACK ARM EXTENSIONS—Extend both arms front (hold), then lower arms to side of body and reach backward (hold), then back and forth, four times.

B. LATERAL ARM LIFTS— Extend both arms up (hold), lower to the side of body with arms straight (hold), then up and down (flapping movement), four times.

C. ARM ROTATIONS—Make a backward circular move-ment with both arms four times, followed by a forward move-ment, four times in each direction.

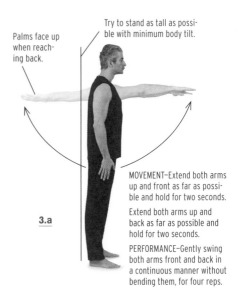

Palms face up when reach-ing back.

Try to stand as tall as possi-ble with minimum body tilt.

3.a

MOVEMENT–Extend both arms up and front as far as possi-ble and hold for two seconds.

Extend both arms up and back as far as possible and hold for two seconds.

PERFORMANCE–Gently swing both arms front and back in a continuous manner without bending them, for four reps.

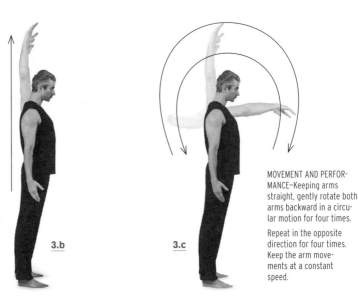

MOVEMENT–Keep both arms straight and keep them as high as possible, holding at top for two seconds and then lower.

Bring both arms up in a flapping manner with arms straight and next to the body.

PERFORMANCE–Gently bring them up and down in a continuous manner for four times.

Only hold for the first time.

3.b

3.c

MOVEMENT AND PERFOR-MANCE–Keeping arms straight, gently rotate both arms backward in a circu-lar motion for four times.

Repeat in the opposite direction for four times. Keep the arm move-ments at a constant speed.

4. HIP ROTATIONS (core)
Start Position—Stand upright with feet shoulder width apart and arms by your sides.
Breathing—Breathe normally.

A. FRONT/BACK PELVIC TILTS—Push the pelvic area backward (hold), then forward (hold), then back and forth, four times.

B. SIDE TO SIDE PELVIC TILTS—Lean pelvic area to right (hold), and left (hold), then side to side, four times.

C. HIP ROTATIONS—Complete a full hip rotation to the left, and then to the right, four times.

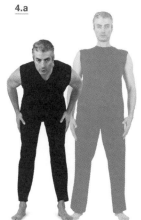

4.a

MOVEMENT—From a standing position, tilt forward slightly while holding your pelvic area backward and hold for two seconds. Push your pelvic area forward as far as you can and hold for two seconds. (Slight arch in the back).

PERFORMANCE—Gently tilt back and forth in a continuous manner for four times.

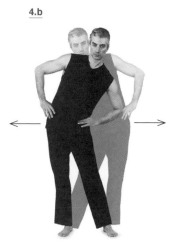

4.b

MOVEMENT—Keeping your body upright, push your pelvis out to one side and hold for two seconds. Repeat on the other side.

PERFORMANCE—Push your pelvic area from one side to the other in a smooth, continuous manner for four reps.

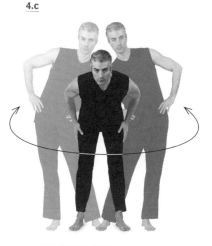

4.c

MOVEMENT AND PERFORMANCE—Gently rotate your pelvic area in a smooth circular motion in one direction, then repeat in the other direction. Alternate directions a total of four times.

5. **FRONT AND BACK LEG COMBO STRETCH** (hamstrings, calves, and groin muscles)
Stand with the feet spread one-and-a-half shoulders in width, with the front foot facing forward (aligned with the body) and rear foot facing sideways.

A. GROIN MUSCLE STRETCH—Lean onto your left leg, stretching the groin muscle of the right leg. Keep body upright

B. HAMSTRING AND CALF STRETCH—Lean back on the right leg, stretching the hamstring and calf muscles of the left leg. Use arms for support

C. FRONT AND BACK LEG COMBO STRETCH—Move back and forth four times, then repeat the stretch on the other side.

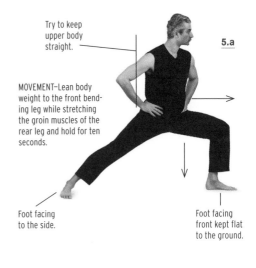

Try to keep upper body straight.

5.a

MOVEMENT–Lean body weight to the front bending leg while stretching the groin muscles of the rear leg and hold for ten seconds.

Foot facing to the side.

Foot facing front kept flat to the ground.

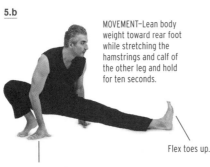

5.b

MOVEMENT–Lean body weight toward rear foot while stretching the hamstrings and calf of the other leg and hold for ten seconds.

Flex toes up.

For better stability, place hands on the floor.

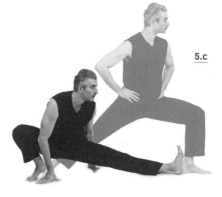

5.c

PERFORMANCE–Combine both stretches; first the groin muscle stretch followed immediately by the hamstring and calf stretch. Repeat four times before starting on the other side.

6. FULL BODY STRETCH (upper body, back, and hamstrings) ’
    Using a wall, chair, or table, stand an arm's distance from the
    chair with legs slightly more than shoulder width apart.

    A. Bend the body as close to parallel with the floor and lean
       buttocks backward, stretching the entire back region (hold).
       Keep legs straight.
    B. Now straighten body, leaning the pelvic area forward while
       arching neck and back area (hold), then gently sway back and
       forth four times.

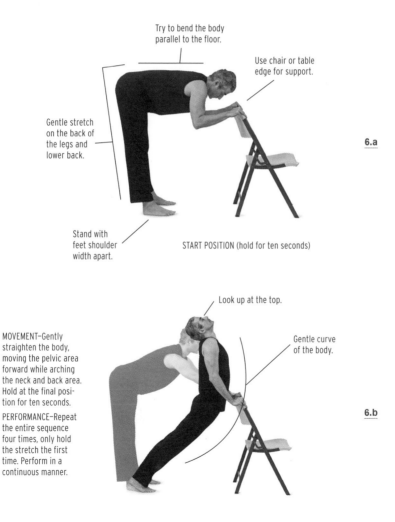

Try to bend the body parallel to the floor.

Use chair or table edge for support.

Gentle stretch on the back of the legs and lower back.

6.a

Stand with feet shoulder width apart.

START POSITION (hold for ten seconds)

Look up at the top.

MOVEMENT–Gently straighten the body, moving the pelvic area forward while arching the neck and back area. Hold at the final position for ten seconds.

PERFORMANCE–Repeat the entire sequence four times, only hold the stretch the first time. Perform in a continuous manner.

Gentle curve of the body.

6.b

FOUNDATION FLOOR STRETCHES

1. **SEATED FLOOR STRETCHES** (hamstrings, calves, groin muscles, and lower back)

    A. SEATED HAMSTRING AND CALF STRETCH—Sit upright with both legs straight and together. Reach both hands toward your feet, repeating four times.

    B. SEATED SINGLE LEG HAMSTRING AND CALF STRETCH— Extend one leg straight and bend the other leg, tucking it on the inside of the straight leg. Lean body and arms toward the extended leg (hold), then return to upright position; repeat four times. Repeat with the other leg. Keep ankles and toes flexed back.

    C. SPREAD EAGLE SIDE REACHES—Sit with legs extended and parted as wide as possible, but without too much discomfort. Lean body with right arm to right leg (hold), then lean to the left (hold), then left and right, for a total of eight times.

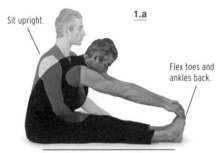

Sit upright.

1.a

Flex toes and ankles back.

Keep both legs straight.

START POSITION—Keep both legs straight and together.

MOVEMENT—Extend both arms and grab your feet with your hands and hold for ten seconds.

PERFORMANCE—Gently repeat the exercise four times, only holding once at the beginning.

BREATHING—Exhale when reaching forward.

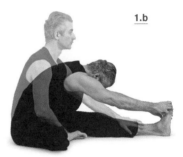

1.b

START POSITION—Keep one leg straight while bending and tucking the other leg.

MOVEMENT—Grab the foot of the straight leg with both hands and hold for ten seconds.

PERFORMANCE—Repeat for a total of four times, then perform on the other leg four times.

BREATHING—Exhale when reaching forward.

START POSITION—Sit upright with legs as far apart as possible.

MOVEMENT—Reach with the same arm to the same leg and hold for ten seconds, then repeat on the other side.

PERFORMANCE—Go from one side to the other eight times.

BREATHING—Exhale when exerting pressure.

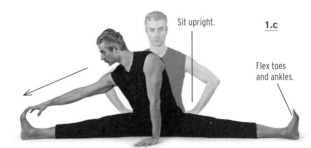

Sit upright.

1.c

Flex toes and ankles.

Keep both legs straight.

D. SPREAD EAGLE CROSSOVERS—In the spread eagle pose keep legs in same position while reaching toward right leg with left arm (hold), then right arm toward left leg (hold), and back and forth, repeating eight times.

E. SPREAD EAGLE PUSH-UPS—Place both hands shoulder-width apart on the floor in front of you, lean your body forward while bending both arms (hold), then lift your body up and down while bending your arms as if you were doing a push-up. Repeat eight times.

1.d

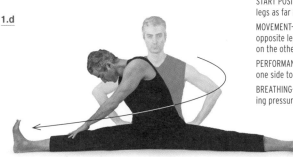

START POSITION–Sit upright with legs as far apart as possible.

MOVEMENT–Try to reach for your opposite leg and hold, then repeat on the other side.

PERFORMANCE–Cross over from one side to the other eight times.

BREATHING–Exhale when exerting pressure.

1.e

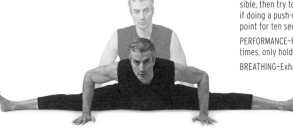

START POSITION–Sit upright with legs as far apart as possible.

MOVEMENT–Place both hands on the floor while keeping your body as upright as possible, then try to lower your upper body as if doing a push-up, holding at the lowest point for ten seconds.

PERFORMANCE–Repeat the sequence eight times, only holding once in the beginning.

BREATHING–Exhale when exerting pressure.

2. **LYING BACK BENT KNEE FLOOR STRETCHES** (core, lower back, and hips)

    A. DOUBLE KNEE BENDS—Lying on your back with knees bent and feet on the floor, bring both knees to the chest, squeeze and hold; then lower legs. Repeat four times.

    B. ALTERNATING SINGLE KNEE BENDS—Lying on your back, bring one knee up to the chest and hold while extending other leg straight along the floor, then switch legs. Repeat four times.

    C. BENT KNEE REVERSE SPLITS—Lying on your back with knees up and together, gently part your knees to stretch and hold. Repeat four times.

2.a

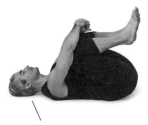

Keep head on the floor.

START POSITION–Lying on your back, bring both knees to your chest while holding them with both hands.

MOVEMENT–Squeeze and hold for ten seconds.

PERFORMANCE–Repeat the sequence four times.

BREATHING–Exhale when squeezing legs.

2.b

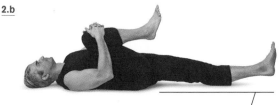

Extend leg, keeping it flexed at the ankle and toes.

START POSITION–Lying back, bring up one knee while extending the other leg.

MOVEMENT–Squeeze and pull the bending leg as high as possible, then switch legs.

PERFORMANCE–Repeat for four reps.

BREATHING–Exhale when squeezing the bending leg.

2.c

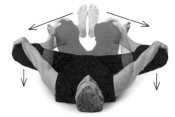

START POSITION–Lie on your back. bringing both knees and feet up

MOVEMENT–Gently part your knees as low as possible and hold for ten seconds.

PERFORMANCE–Repeat four times.

BREATHING–Exhale when parting the knees.

D. DOUBLE KNEE TWISTS—Lying on your back with legs bent together and feet on the floor, gently lower both knees to the left side of the floor (hold), then to the right side (hold), then move side-to-side. Repeat four times. Make sure not to lift the arms off the floor.

E. SINGLE KNEE TWISTS—Lying on your back, bend one leg with foot on the floor, take other leg and cross over the leg on the floor, then from that position gently twist the lower body side-to-side. Repeat four times. Repeat with other leg on top.

2.d

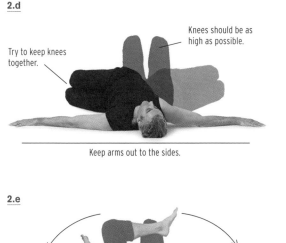

Knees should be as high as possible.

Try to keep knees together.

Keep arms out to the sides.

START POSITION–Lie on your back with both feet on the floor and knees bent.

MOVEMENT–While lying back, gently lower both bent legs to one side, holding the first time for ten seconds on both sides.

PERFORMANCE–Alternate from one side to the other for four times.

BREATHING–Exhale when lowering knees to the side.

2.e

START POSITION–Lying on your back, bend one knee, keeping the foot on the floor, then cross the floor leg with the other leg.

MOVEMENT–While keeping the legs in that position, try to lower both legs, twisting at the hips.

PERFORMANCE–Hold at each end position for a few seconds, then go back and forth four times. Repeat with the other leg.

BREATHING–Exhale when lowering the legs to the side.

Eating Plan Week 1: White Belt Beginner Level

Eating for Week 1

Don't change your eating pattern. Consume your normal meals.

In week 1, I want you to really increase your liquid intake.

Try your best to drink at least four (8 oz) glasses of water per day from now on. Water will be very important to this eating plan. Think of water as your new best friend.

You can continue drinking your morning coffee, just don't go crazy with the sugar or sweeteners. Like I said, this will be a very gradual change. You don't have to quit anything.

I'm sure you've heard or read that you should drink at least eight glasses of water a day. I don't know about you but some days, it's hard for me to drink that much water. At the beginning, a more manageable goal would be at least four glasses a day.

If you are still thirsty after four glasses, by all means, drink more water. I think using smaller water bottles or containers work the best to help you keep track. For example, if you use 16-oz water bottles, drink 2 bottles and that will be equivalent to 4 glasses.

YELLOW BELT BEGINNER LEVEL (WEEK TWO)– KEEP IT GOING

You're moving in the right direction, and not losing focus is key at this level. You might be saying either of two things at this stage:

- I don't know if this regimen is going to get me to where I want to be.
     or
- If this is going to get me in shape, it's a piece of cake!

I'm hoping that you're thinking the second way. Exercising and getting into shape should feel easy and somewhat fun. That's why it's important to do it gradually with an open-minded attitude. Keep reminding yourself that working out is not a temporary fix, so that when you get to where you want to be, that's not the end. Instead, think of it as one of the necessities in life for health, happiness, and longevity.

At this stage, it's important to maintain the same course of exercise routines as the white belt stage, but slightly step it up a notch. This means that you have to start putting some emphasis on the pace of your workouts.

Strengthening Plan Week 2: Yellow Belt Beginner Level

Strength goals:
1. This week we're going to continue working with our fundamental calisthenic exercises—our foundation—from the previous week,

but we're going to step it up a notch by increasing the minimum time duration for each routine to 45 seconds (of course 60 seconds is still our goal), and with very little rest in-between the exercises.
2. Make sure to practice proper form and technique, while trying to get that pumped feeling of the muscles being worked on.
3. Perform three days this week.

1. PUSH-UPS (45–60 seconds)
2. LEG SQUATS (45–60 seconds)
3. LYING BACK BENT LEG LIFTS (45–60 seconds)

Stretching Plan Week 2: Yellow Belt Beginner Level

Stretching goals:
1. Perform standing foundation stretches daily when waking up. Just like washing your face or brushing your teeth, these exercises should be part of your everyday routine. Regarding floor stretches, do them at least three days this week.
2. It's not how fast you do the stretches—it's using the proper technique that's important. The slower and deeper your stretches are, the more your body will benefit. In addition, it is essential that your breathing be synchronized to your stretching rhythm to prevent injuries.

Eating Plan Week 2: Yellow Belt Beginner Level GET READY TO CHALLENGE YOURSELF!

Continue the same water intake regimen as week 1, but this week, aim for at least six glasses of water a day. Remember, consumption of water is key.

As for your food intake, eat normally for breakfast and lunch.

But for dinner, you're going to try something different: only eat three-quarters of what you used to eat.

Now that dinner will be smaller than you're accustomed to, I want you to include a healthy light snack before dinner. It can be fruit, low-fat yogurt, a simple salad, nuts, or something healthy to curb your appetite until dinner. This way, you will be reducing the amount of calories you take in without it being such a drastic shock to the body.

If you're still feeling hungry after dinner, drink more water. Whatever you do, avoid snacking—the tendency after eating dinner is to have something that will satisfy the craving for dessert, like cake or pie. If you're a big soda or juice drinker, try to to limit how much soda or juice you drink. A 12 oz can of soda contains 140 calories. If you have a can of soda with lunch and another for dinner, just by eliminating those two cans of soda every day, you would lose 30 pounds in a year! The more sweetened drinks you eliminate, the more weight you stand to lose. As an overweight teenager, I used to drink two cans of soda a day. As soon as I replaced my soda consumption with water, the weight came off.

Believe it or not, juice actually contains more calories than soda: about 120 calories for an 8 oz cup. If you absolutely have to drink juice, I recommend investing in a juicer and making your own homemade juice. Not only is this a lot healthier but you can be sure there is no added sugar or artificial flavors.

If soda or juice is something you are having difficulty giving up, try to limit yourself to one for the entire day. Then one every other day and so on, until you can totally eliminate it. Try to drink soft drinks from bottles if possible, instead of cans. The mentality of most people who drink from cans is to finish the whole thing in one sitting. With bottles, it's much easier to drink a little bit, screw the lid back on and save the rest for later.

This week, I also want you to start reducing your fat calorie intake. This means less fried foods or foods with high saturated fat content or high cholesterol. Again, if you've always had these foods as part of your daily consumption, eat it in limited quantities earlier in the day.

Michael's Thoughts on Being a Beginner

When I first started as a white belt, I had many fears about working out. My main fear was that I couldn't hack it. My fear was that my endurance and stamina were shot because when you're smoking, basically you don't breathe. My other fear was probably a bigger concern—that I wouldn't stick with it. Like I said, I've tried a lot of fitness clubs and gyms. I even joined a dance class when I was much younger, I think I went once. I joined a martial arts place 12 years ago, about a year or so before I came to Grandmaster Kang. I really liked the instructor and I was all psyched, but I never went. I think I paid the initiation fee and I never went once. I was just afraid to fail and something kept me from going.

I worried that I wasn't going to be able to succeed. I've been training with

Grandmaster for 10 years now and I've seen people from all walks of life, all ages, in all states of physical health, some people come in and they're quite overweight when they start. I admire them. It's hard to show up at a gym or somewhere where most people are fit and doing these amazing martial arts moves and you come in and you're overweight and you're a white belt. That takes a lot of guts. I've seen them stick with it and succeed, and progress.

I got over that fear. Martial arts is something that I always wanted to do since I was a kid, but for some reason there was a block, like I felt I couldn't succeed in it. Probably because I never found the right teacher.

Fitness and health are a gift, a very, very valuable gift that you can give to yourself and your family. My advice is to find something that's challenging in a good way. I'm very biased—my advice is to do martial arts! I'll come out and say it! And why? Because in martial arts, you're learning a skill, and that's interesting. To have to pursue learning the knowledge and pursue perfecting a skill, all the time, is a lot more engaging and keeps your interest a lot longer than doing the same repetitive motions week after week, year after year. And you're learning something that has a practical application in the world. Hopefully you'll never have to use it, but knowing that you can defend yourself also helps you become, ironically, a less aggressive person.

Because you're less fearful and more comfortable in your body, you give off less aggressive vibes. When you're a fearful person, I think it triggers aggression, because someone who's aggressive picks up on that. When you're fearful, you're kind of expecting aggression. But when you're not so fearful, you're tuning out of that frequency. Martial artists, really, really good martial artists, they're the least aggressive types of people I've ever met. Actually, they're some of the kindest, most pleasant people I know.

My advice is to try martial arts, but the important thing is to find the right teacher. I think many martial arts disciplines are very good (I'm sure they all have their benefits), but the important thing is the teacher. You have to have somebody who you can really put trust in, who has a lot of integrity, who really stresses the tenets. It's not just about being the best fighter or kicking the highest or being a sparring champion. It's really about challenging yourself to do the best you can do. If people are resistant and they're a little afraid to come, I tell them it's not about competition. My son does little league—now that's competition! It's more competitive in the little leagues than martial arts because in martial arts you're really only challenging yourself. You're not trying to win. The overarching emphasis is on improving yourself.

I had zero flexibility when I first started. I mean, really, there was no flexibility. After a not-terribly-long period of time, I was amazed at what I could start doing. I think the tightness in your body is a metaphor for the tightness in your mind and tightness in your spirit. With Taekwondo, I believe flexibility is a good measure of your progress. And as you progress through the belt levels, if you're training properly, your flexibility's going to increase.

Where I'm at now with my flexibility in comparison to where I started is like comparing night and day. I'm almost 50 and started very late: I don't know if I'll ever be able to do full splits on the floor, but with my side splits, I come pretty close. My legs were much more like an equilateral triangle when I started and now the angle's become much more obtuse. Working on flexibility and stretches is a great release of tension. I think we store a lot of negative emotion and tension in our muscles, and stretching just releases a lot of that, it releases a lot of pent up energy. Stretching is complementary to breathing, and will greatly improve your technique.

GREEN BELT INTERMEDIATE LEVEL (WEEK THREE)— DON'T LOSE FOCUS

This level is a good measure of your progress, since it takes 21 days to make something habit forming, and by the week's end you will have reached that time. The concept here is to develop the right habits that will give you the confidence to continue on your journey.

Strengthening Plan Week 3: Green Belt Intermediate Level

Strength goals:
1. Perform the previous level exercises (fundamental calisthenics) for at least 60 seconds as a warm-up.
2. Incorporate the use of light dumbbell weights to increase the strength and definition to your shoulders, back, triceps, and biceps. These dumbbell exercises should be performed for 30–60 seconds per each routine, with no rest in-between.
3. You can repeat the sequence or use heavier weights, depending on your personal fitness level.
4. Perform three days this week.

1. PUSH-UPS (60 seconds)

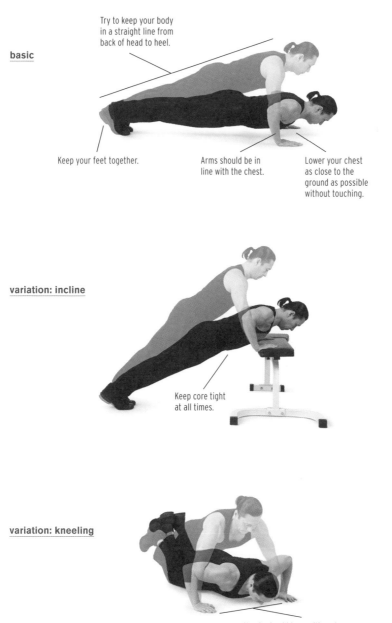

basic

Try to keep your body in a straight line from back of head to heel.

Keep your feet together.

Arms should be in line with the chest.

Lower your chest as close to the ground as possible without touching.

variation: incline

Keep core tight at all times.

variation: kneeling

Hands should be positioned slightly wider than the chest.

2. LEG SQUATS (60 seconds)

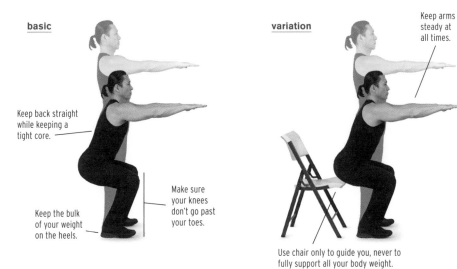

basic

variation

Keep back straight while keeping a tight core.

Keep the bulk of your weight on the heels.

Make sure your knees don't go past your toes.

Keep arms steady at all times.

Use chair only to guide you, never to fully support all your body weight.

3. LYING BACK BENT LEG LIFTS (60 seconds)

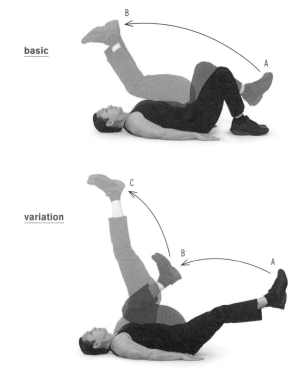

basic

B

A

variation

C

B

A

4. REVERSE BACK ROWS (30–60 seconds)

Stand with feet together, knees slightly bent, body tilting forward (approximately 45 degrees). Extend both arms so they are parallel to the upper part of your legs. Lift both arms, pulling and lifting the elbows up and back, bringing the hands in line with the chest (hold).

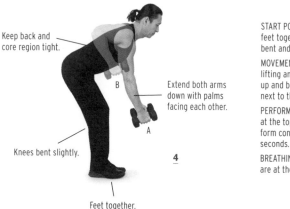

Keep back and core region tight.

B

Knees bent slightly.

Feet together.

Extend both arms down with palms facing each other.

A

4

START POSITION–Stand with feet together, knees slightly bent and body tilted forward.

MOVEMENT–Lift both arms, lifting and pulling the elbows up and back, bringing hands next to the chest.

PERFORMANCE–Hold slightly at the top of the move, perform continuously for 30-60 seconds.

BREATHING–Inhale when arms are at the highest position.

5. SHOULDER LATERAL LIFTS (30–60 seconds)

Stand or sit upright with arms extended. Keeping both arms straight, lift to shoulder height (hold), then lower. Keep palms facing down.

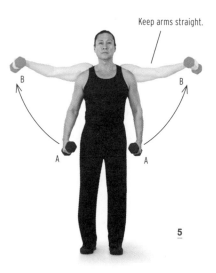

Keep arms straight.

B

B

A

A

5

START POSITION–Stand tall with feet shoulder width apart with arms by your sides.

MOVEMENT–While keeping both arms straight, lift them sideways in a smooth controlled manner to shoulder level, holding slightly at the top, then lower.

PERFORMANCE–Perform continuously for 30-60 seconds.

BREATHING–Inhale when lifting both arms.

6. TRICEP KICKBACKS (30–60 seconds)

Standing in the same pose as in the back row exercises, with arms bent against the body lift both elbows as high as possible. Keeping arms in that position, extend both arms back and up, with the pinky part of the hand being at the highest point. Do not swing the arms.

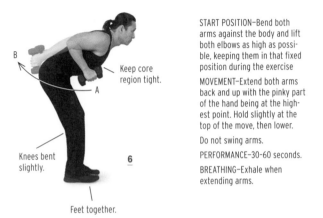

Keep core region tight.

Knees bent slightly.

6

Feet together.

START POSITION–Bend both arms against the body and lift both elbows as high as possible, keeping them in that fixed position during the exercise

MOVEMENT–Extend both arms back and up with the pinky part of the hand being at the highest point. Hold slightly at the top of the move, then lower.

Do not swing arms.

PERFORMANCE–30-60 seconds.

BREATHING–Exhale when extending arms.

7. BICEP CURLS (30–60 seconds)

Standing upright, extend both arms down next to the body with palms facing inward. Bend both arms while lifting hands to shoulder height and turn palms to face the body (hold), then lower arms while trying to prevent the arms from swinging.

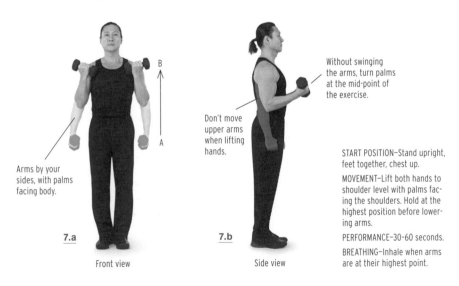

Arms by your sides, with palms facing body.

Don't move upper arms when lifting hands.

Without swinging the arms, turn palms at the mid-point of the exercise.

7.a

Front view

7.b

Side view

START POSITION–Stand upright, feet together, chest up.

MOVEMENT–Lift both hands to shoulder level with palms facing the shoulders. Hold at the highest position before lowering arms.

PERFORMANCE–30-60 seconds.

BREATHING–Inhale when arms are at their highest point.

Stretching Plan Week 3: Green Belt Intermediate Level

Stretching goals:

1. In addition to standing foundation stretches, work on a combination stretching routines to work the entire body.
2. Learn some basic Taekwondo stretching kicks.
3. Add more floor stretches to the previous level and combine them at the end.
4. Perform three days this week.

1. STANDING FOUNDATION STRETCHES (white/yellow level)
    1. Neck stretches

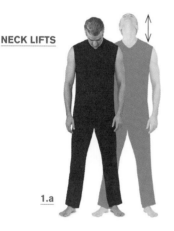

NECK LIFTS

1.a

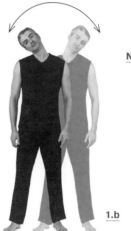

NECK TILTS

1.b

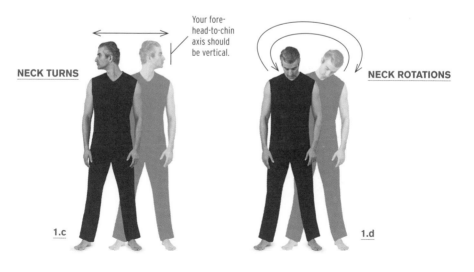

NECK TURNS

Your forehead-to-chin axis should be vertical.

1.c

NECK ROTATIONS

1.d

2. Shoulder stretches

UP / DOWN SHRUGS

Hold and squeeze at the highest point for two seconds.

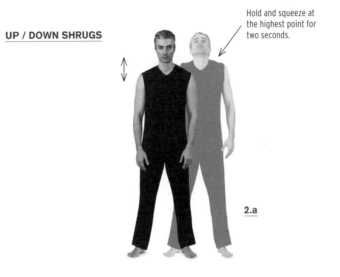

2.a

FRONT / BACK SHRUGS

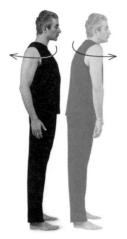

2.b

SHOULDER ROTATIONS

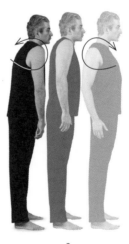

2.c

3. Arm stretches

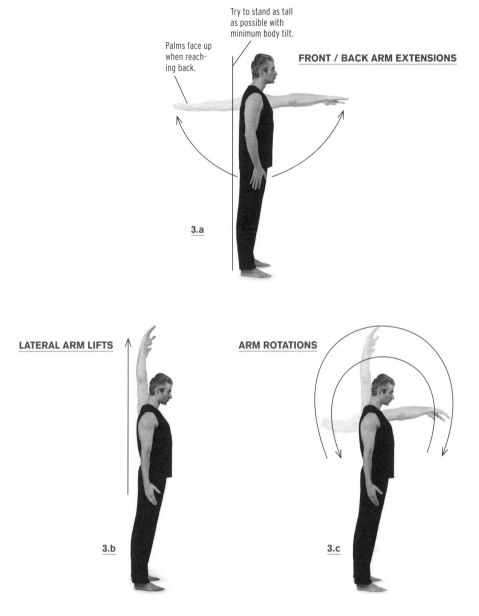

Try to stand as tall as possible with minimum body tilt.

Palms face up when reaching back.

FRONT / BACK ARM EXTENSIONS

3.a

LATERAL ARM LIFTS

3.b

ARM ROTATIONS

3.c

4. Hip/pelvis stretches

FRONT / BACK PELVIC TILTS

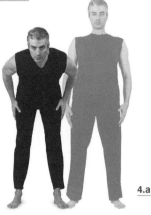

4.a

SIDE-TO-SIDE PELVIC TILTS

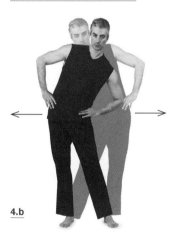

4.b

HIP ROTATIONS

4.c

5. Front and back leg combo stretches

GROIN MUSCLE STRETCH

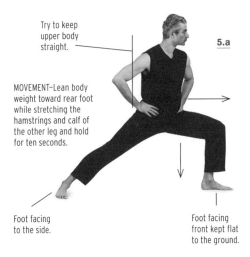

Try to keep upper body straight.

5.a

MOVEMENT—Lean body weight toward rear foot while stretching the hamstrings and calf of the other leg and hold for ten seconds.

Foot facing to the side.

Foot facing front kept flat to the ground.

HAMSTRING AND CALF STRETCH

FRONT AND BACK LEG COMBO STRETCH

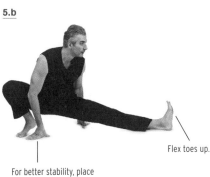

5.b

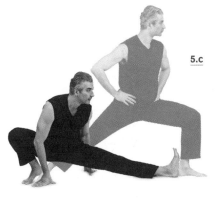

5.c

Flex toes up.

For better stability, place hands on the floor.

6. Full body stretch

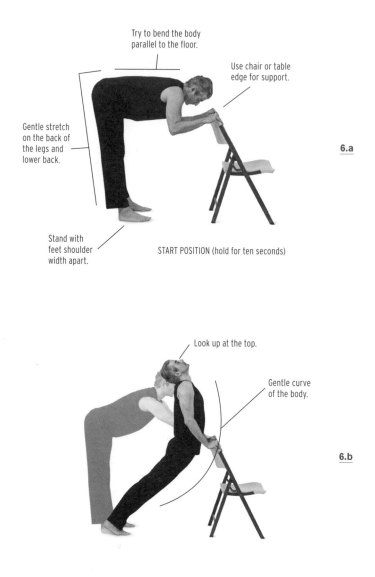

Try to bend the body parallel to the floor.

Use chair or table edge for support.

Gentle stretch on the back of the legs and lower back.

6.a

Stand with feet shoulder width apart.

START POSITION (hold for ten seconds)

Look up at the top.

Gentle curve of the body.

6.b

2. **ALTERNATING ARM EXTENSIONS** (arms, upper body, hamstrings)
   A. UP AND DOWN—Lift one arm up while lowering other arm, then switch arms, alternating arms eight times.

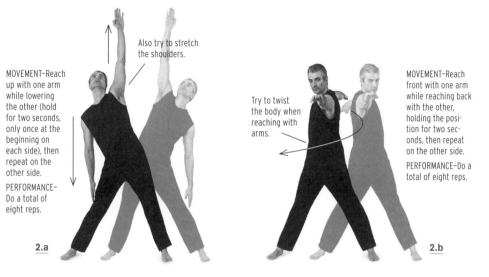

Also try to stretch the shoulders.

MOVEMENT—Reach up with one arm while lowering the other (hold for two seconds, only once at the beginning on each side), then repeat on the other side.

PERFORMANCE—Do a total of eight reps.

2.a

Try to twist the body when reaching with arms.

MOVEMENT—Reach front with one arm while reaching back with the other, holding the position for two seconds, then repeat on the other side.

PERFORMANCE—Do a total of eight reps.

2.b

   B. FRONT AND BACK—Extend one arm front and the other back, switching eight times.
   C. SIDE TO SIDE—Reach the left hand to the right side of the body and the right hand to left side, while rotating upper body; switch eight times.
   D. CRISS CROSS—With feet spread double shoulder width, twist upper body downward while reaching to right leg with left arm and extending right arm up. Then switch arms positions leg while maintaining a bent over position. Repeat eight times.

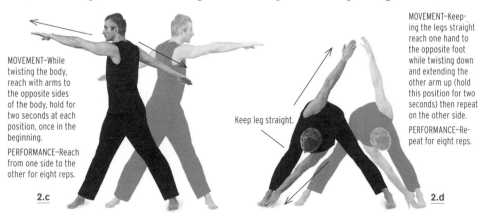

MOVEMENT—While twisting the body, reach with arms to the opposite sides of the body, hold for two seconds at each position, once in the beginning.

PERFORMANCE—Reach from one side to the other for eight reps.

2.c

Keep leg straight.

MOVEMENT—Keeping the legs straight reach one hand to the opposite foot while twisting down and extending the other arm up (hold this position for two seconds) then repeat on the other side.

PERFORMANCE—Repeat for eight reps.

2.d

3. **KNEE KICKS WITH CHAIR** (core and hips)
Stand next to a chair, holding the back part with the supporting leg closest to the chair.

Start Position—Stand tall with feet close together using chair. (When doing the four reps you can touch or not touch the floor when lowering the stretching leg.)

Breathing—Exhale gently when lifting the leg.

A. Perform a straight up knee kick with the non supporting leg, repeat four times each leg.
B. Kick knee to the opposite shoulder (across the body).
C. Kick knee outward from the same shoulder.
D. Perform outside circular knee kicks.
E. Perform inside circular knee kicks.

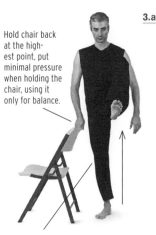

3.a

Hold chair back at the highest point, put minimal pressure when holding the chair, using it only for balance.

MOVEMENT–Bring the non-supported knee up and down

PERFORMANCE–Do four reps on one leg, then repeat on the other leg.

Standing leg should be closest to the chair.

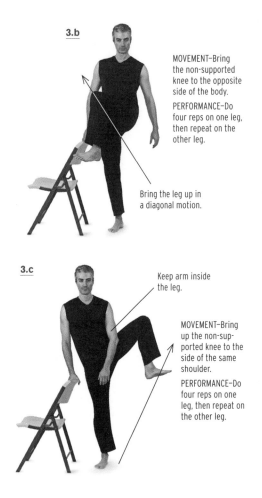

3.b

MOVEMENT–Bring the non-supported knee to the opposite side of the body.

PERFORMANCE–Do four reps on one leg, then repeat on the other leg.

Bring the leg up in a diagonal motion.

3.c

Keep arm inside the leg.

MOVEMENT–Bring up the non-supported knee to the side of the same shoulder.

PERFORMANCE–Do four reps on one leg, then repeat on the other leg.

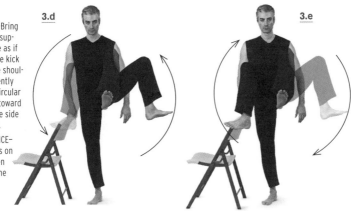

MOVEMENT–Bring up the non-supported knee as if doing a knee kick to the same shoulder, then gently execute a circular movement toward the opposite side of the body.

PERFORMANCE–Do four reps on one leg, then repeat on the other leg.

3.d

3.e

MOVEMENT–Bring up the non-supported knee as if doing an opposite-shoulder knee kick, then gently execute a circular movement toward the outside of the body. Keep the move smooth and continuous, while emphasizing the hip rotation.

PERFORMANCE–Do four reps on one leg, then repeat on the other leg.

4. **STRAIGHT LEG STRETCHES WITH CHAIR** (core, hips, and legs)
   Hold the chair on the high back portion with the closest hand and inside leg supporting your body weight. Always bring back the stretching leg to the starting point.

   Breathing—Exhale when lifting the kicking leg.

   Start Position—Hold chair back at the highest point, putting minimal hand pressure.

   A. STRAIGHT LEG FRONT KICK—Supporting body weight with right leg, bring the left leg up and down in a straight position without tilting the body, four times. Repeat on other leg.

   B. OPPOSITE SHOULDER FRONT KICK—Lift left leg diagonally across body to the right side and back down, four times. Repeat on other leg.

   C. SAME SHOULDER FRONT KICK—Lift left leg diagonally to the outside of the body while keeping left arm down, four times. Repeat on other leg.

   D. OUTSIDE CIRCULAR STRAIGHT LEG KICK—Perform an outer circular motion kick with left leg straight, keeping left arm up, four times. Repeat on other leg.

   E. INSIDE CIRCULAR STRAIGHT LEG KICK—Execute an inner circular motion kick with left leg straight, keeping left arm up, four times. Repeat on other leg.

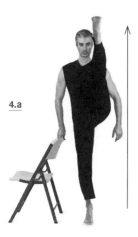

4.a

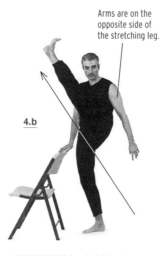

4.b

Arms are on the opposite side of the stretching leg.

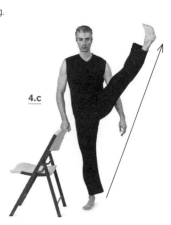

4.c

MOVEMENT–Keeping the non-supporting leg straight, bring it up in a smooth controlled manner, minimizing any excess movement.

PERFORMANCE–Do four reps on one leg, then switch legs.

MOVEMENT–With leg straight and body facing front, bring the stretching leg up toward the opposite side of the body as if drawing an upward diagonal line.

PERFORMANCE–Do four reps on one leg, then four reps on the other leg.

Keep arm to the side to prevent over-turning the upper body.

MOVEMENT–Lift the stretching leg in a diagonal motion toward the same shoulder.

PERFORMANCE–Do four reps on each leg.

4.d

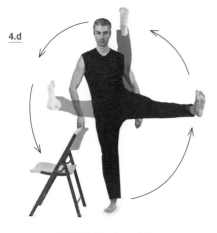

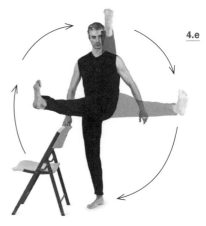

4.e

MOVEMENT–Bring the stretching leg to the outside of the same shoulder, then gently circle it up and around to the other side of the body.

PERFORMANCE–Do four reps on each leg.

MOVEMENT–Bring the stretching leg to the opposite side of the body, then gently circle the leg up and around to the other side of the body, executing in a smooth continuous manner.

PERFORMANCE–Do four reps on one leg, then repeat on the other leg.

5. SEATED FOUNDATION FLOOR STRETCHES (white/yellow level)

SEATED HAMSTRING AND CALF STRETCH

SEATED SINGLE LEG HAMSTRING AND CALF STRETCH

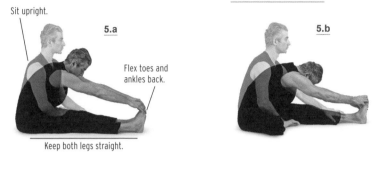

Sit upright.

5.a

Flex toes and ankles back.

Keep both legs straight.

5.b

SPREAD EAGLE SIDE REACHES

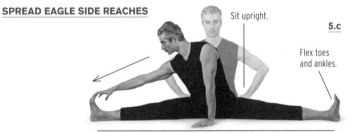

Sit upright.

5.c

Flex toes and ankles.

Keep both legs straight.

SPREAD EAGLE CROSSOVERS

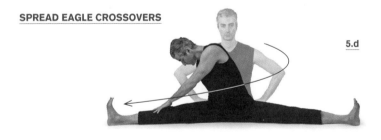

5.d

SPREAD EAGLE PUSH-UPS

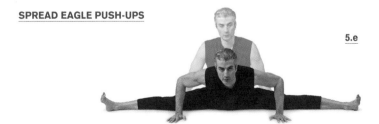

5.e

6. LYING BACK FOUNDATION BENT KNEE FLOOR STRETCHES

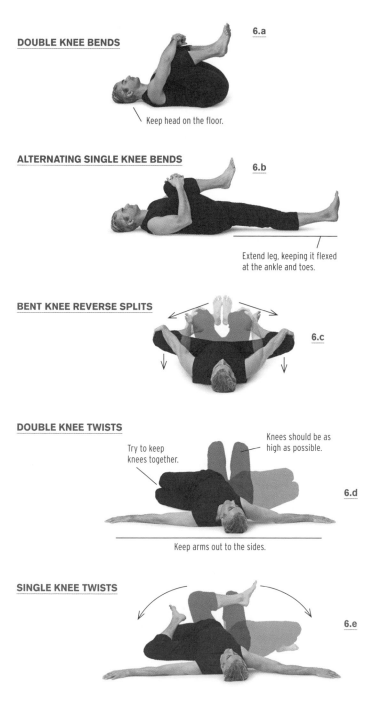

DOUBLE KNEE BENDS

6.a

Keep head on the floor.

ALTERNATING SINGLE KNEE BENDS

6.b

Extend leg, keeping it flexed at the ankle and toes.

BENT KNEE REVERSE SPLITS

6.c

DOUBLE KNEE TWISTS

Try to keep knees together.

Knees should be as high as possible.

6.d

Keep arms out to the sides.

SINGLE KNEE TWISTS

6.e

7. LYING BACK STRAIGHT LEG FLOOR STRETCHES

   A. BOTH LEGS—Lying on your back, bring both knees to the chest, then slowly extend them straight upward while holding on to the back of the legs with your hands (hold). Repeat four times.

   B. SINGLE LEG—Lying on your back, grip behind the knee of the right leg while extending it straight up, at the same time lowering the left leg to the ground (or slightly off the floor, depending on flexibility), then switch legs. Repeat four times.

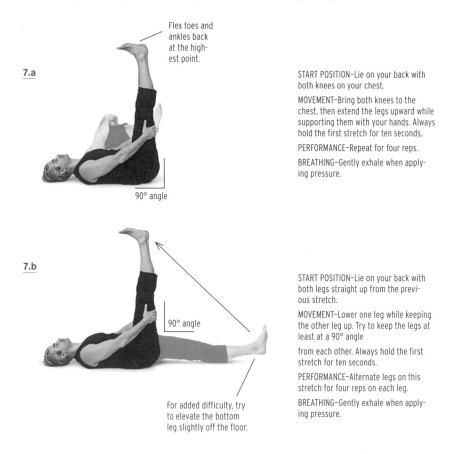

7.a

Flex toes and ankles back at the highest point.

90° angle

START POSITION—Lie on your back with both knees on your chest.

MOVEMENT—Bring both knees to the chest, then extend the legs upward while supporting them with your hands. Always hold the first stretch for ten seconds.

PERFORMANCE—Repeat for four reps.

BREATHING—Gently exhale when applying pressure.

7.b

90° angle

For added difficulty, try to elevate the bottom leg slightly off the floor.

START POSITION—Lie on your back with both legs straight up from the previous stretch.

MOVEMENT—Lower one leg while keeping the other leg up. Try to keep the legs at least at a 90° angle

from each other. Always hold the first stretch for ten seconds.

PERFORMANCE—Alternate legs on this stretch for four reps on each leg.

BREATHING—Gently exhale when applying pressure.

   C. REVERSE SPREAD EAGLE—Lying on your back with both legs extended upward, gently part the legs to opposite sides, using your hands to hold. Repeat four times.

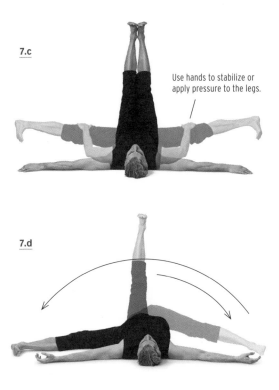

7.c

Use hands to stabilize or apply pressure to the legs.

START POSITION–Lie on your back with both legs straight up. (Try to have both legs up at a 90° angle off the floor.)

MOVEMENT–Gently part the legs to the opposite sides. Always hold the first stretch for ten seconds.

PERFORMANCE–Repeat four reps.

BREATHING–Gently exhale when applying pressure.

7.d

START POSITION–Lie on your back with both legs straight on the floor with arms out to the sides (human-cross position).

MOVEMENT–Lift left leg up as high as possible, then lower it to the right hand, then bring it back up to the top and lower toward the left hand.

PERFORMANCE–Go back and forth (think of your leg as a windshield wiper blade) for four times, then repeat with the right leg.

BREATHING–Exhale while lowering the stretching leg toward either side.

D. WIPER BLADE STRETCH—Lying on your back with arms flat out to the sides for support, lift your left leg straight up as high as you can. Gently lower it to the right, then bring it back up to the top and lower the leg toward the left side, repeating four times (think of your leg as a windshield wiper blade). Repeat with other leg.

Note: After doing foundation seated floor stretches, combine all the lying back stretches together, starting from the bent knee stretches to the straight leg stretches.

Eating Plan Week 3: Green Belt Intermediate Level

Continue the same eating plan from week 2. Eat your normal breakfast, lunch, snack and now reduced portion for dinner. Try to drink at least 8 glasses of water!

If the first week of having three-quarters of what you were used to for dinner was difficult, congratulations for making it past that week!

It will get easier as your body gets used to the new portions.

BLUE BELT INTERMEDIATE LEVEL (WEEK FOUR)— DON'T GET TOO COMFORTABLE

All too often when my students reach this level, they get a little lazy. They feel they've mastered all the fundamentals, so they take it easy. This is when I stress to them that they have to wake up and push themselves even harder, otherwise all the effort and progress they've made so far is going to go down the drain.

Sure, sometimes when you do things repetitively, it can seem boring, but this is when you have to stop babying yourself. Take it to the next level by making your workouts more regimented and be a lot more disciplined with your eating habits.

It's always easier to give up or make excuses, but we're talking about your health and your life. Do you really want to give up on that?

Strengthening Plan Week 4: Blue Belt Intermediate Level

Strength goals:
1. Perform the fundamental calisthenics for at least 60 seconds.
2. Repeat the dumbbell exercises from the previous week. By now you should have a certain rhythm to your exercising, meaning you should be able to go from one routine to the next with hardly any rest, performing all exercises for 45–60 seconds.
3. For a greater challenge, either try to do more repetitions within 60 seconds or repeat all the strength training exercises for this level again.
4. Perform three days this week.

1. PUSH-UPS (60 seconds)
2. LEG SQUATS (60 seconds)
3. LYING BACK BENT LEG LIFTS (60 seconds)
4. REVERSE BACK ROWS (45–60 seconds)
5. SHOULDER LATERAL LIFTS (45–60 seconds)
6. TRICEP KICKBACKS (45–60 seconds)
7. BICEP CURLS (45–60 seconds)

Stretching Plan Week 4: Blue Belt Intermediate Level

Stretching goals:
1. Perform all the stretches from the previous level.
2. Try to do all the standing stretching routines at a faster pace, or possibly repeat the sequence for a harder cardio workout.
3. Do the standing foundation stretches daily, and all the other exercises at least three days this week.
4. The only way you'll develop greater flexibility is to understand that each time you stretch, you have to reach farther, meaning you're definitely going to feel a certain level of pressure pain (dull, not sharp) and soreness.

Eating Plan Week 4: Blue Belt Intermediate Level

For week 4, your water consumption isn't going to change. That means still at least 8 glasses per day. If you feel at any time you can totally eliminate sugary beverages, that's excellent, do it.

Your breakfast is going to stay the same, but for lunch, you're going to eat only three-quarters of what you used to eat. Now that lunch is a smaller portion than you are used to, you can add a healthy snack between breakfast and lunch.

For dinner, continue to eat the same reduced-sized portion as week 3. But now it's not really three-quarters of a meal size, it's the new normal size portion. Remember you can have a small snack between lunch and dinner.

Don't forget, it is gradual "slow and steady" that is going to work.

Michael's Thoughts on the Intermediate Level

Intermediate stage is really exciting and fun because now the basic techniques start to become second nature. You don't have to think as much all the time. When you're a beginner, you have to think, "How do I do a side kick? How much do I have to turn?" By the time you're intermediate, you've done a lot of these basics hundreds of times, so your muscle memory starts to be engaged and that's when it starts to get fun. As the forms get more complicated while you move up the belt system, you feel a sense of accomplishment. You also get a sense that you haven't mastered anything yet, of course. I mean, maybe you'll never master anything. But you feel like, okay, I do know how to do this stretch. So when your instructor says, "Throw a hook kick," you know immediately what that is, and your body just does it rather than thinking about each step—you start to develop a little bit of fluidity.

I think intermediate level is also a tricky time because you find out if you really have the perseverance and the dedication. If you do have that dedication—and it's dedication to yourself, above all—then the sky's the limit.

If you look at pictures from the time right before I started and a year later, you'll see a bloated quality that's gone. In the first year I lost a good 10 pounds. And that's from three times a week, sometimes more, sometimes less, but I maintained a three day a week average. Flexibility immediately started to increase. My endurance started to increase. My strength started to increase, my muscle tone got better.

Martial arts really started to lead me toward a healthier lifestyle, because as I started moving through the ranks, I wanted to be better and better. And I couldn't progress doing martial arts if I continued to smoke, and I knew smoking was bad, and this was a real inspiration for me to quit smoking. And I knew if I was abusing my body with bad food and bad diet, and drinking too much and over-indulging in unhealthy food, I couldn't progress as much as I wanted—so I made adjustments there, too.

Martial arts also led me to meditation, which is another Eastern art form of wellness and health. Taekwondo inspired me to it because it definitely takes a certain amount of mental focus and attention to perform martial arts, and it led me to a path where meditation became a part of my life.

BROWN BELT ADVANCED LEVEL (WEEK FIVE)– A NEW AWAKENING

I consider this level the equivalent of getting a "second wind." If you made it this far, you should be very proud of yourself. Achieving this level indicates not just the physical challenges that you've overcome, but also the mental understanding and maturity you've developed about exercising and eating.

Continue to work forward, but don't forget the fundamentals of what you've learned so far. In order to move forward, an understanding of past and present must be worked into the formula.

As already mentioned, this requires a level of maturity where your training has to be very precise—don't leave any screws missing. As for your eating regimen, push yourself a little more. On one of the days, drastically cut your food intake and make your workout more intense. This will be a challenge for mind and body.

Strengthening Plan Week 5: Brown Belt Advanced Level

Strength goals:
1. Perform all the fundamental calisthenics and dumbbell exercises from the previous levels for 30–60 seconds as a warm-up.
2. Incorporate combination leg strengthening exercises done simultaneously with the upper body dumbbell routines. Doing the exercises in this manner will not only increase your cardio workout, but will also keep you totally focused, since every part of your body will be kept busy. Try to perform these exercises for 30–60 seconds each.
3. Perform three days this week.

1. PUSH-UPS (30–60 seconds)

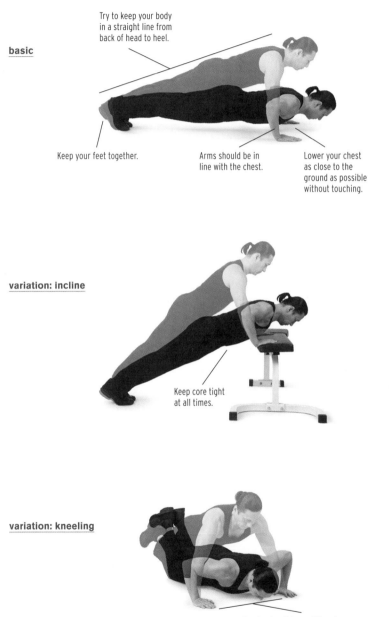

basic

Try to keep your body in a straight line from back of head to heel.

Keep your feet together.

Arms should be in line with the chest.

Lower your chest as close to the ground as possible without touching.

variation: incline

Keep core tight at all times.

variation: kneeling

Hands should be positioned slightly wider than the chest.

2. LEG SQUATS (30–60 seconds)

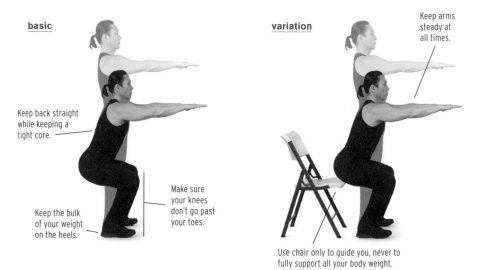

basic

Keep back straight while keeping a tight core.

Keep the bulk of your weight on the heels.

Make sure your knees don't go past your toes.

variation

Keep arms steady at all times.

Use chair only to guide you, never to fully support all your body weight.

3. LYING BACK BENT LEG LIFTS (60 seconds)

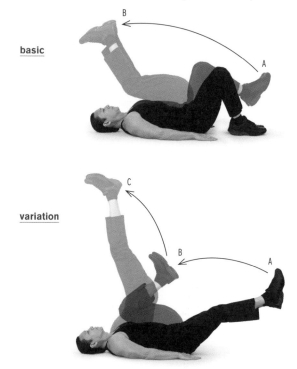

basic

B

A

variation

C

B

A

4. REVERSE BACK ROWS (30–60 seconds)

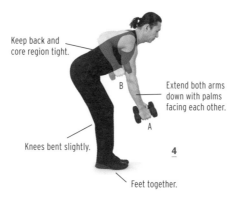

Keep back and core region tight.

Extend both arms down with palms facing each other.

Knees bent slightly.

Feet together.

5. SHOULDER LATERAL LIFTS (30–60 seconds)

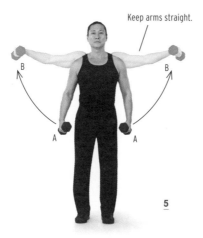

Keep arms straight.

6. TRICEP KICKBACKS (30–60 seconds)

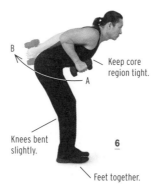

Keep core region tight.

Knees bent slightly.

Feet together.

7. BICEP CURLS (30–60 seconds)

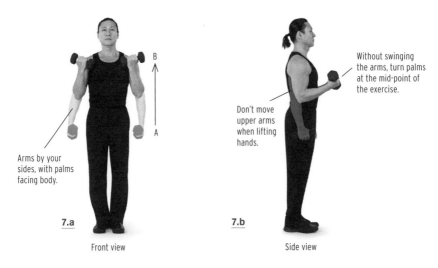

B

↑

A

Arms by your
sides, with palms
facing body.

Don't move
upper arms
when lifting
hands.

Without swinging
the arms, turn palms
at the mid-point of
the exercise.

7.a

Front view

7.b

Side view

8. LATERAL PUSH-UPS (30–60 seconds)

Realign body from left to right, performing a push-up in each position.

basic

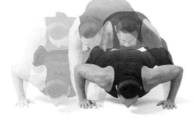

START POSITION–Push-up position with arms and legs spread out wider than shoulders.

MOVEMENT–Perform a push-up, then bring arms and legs together and reposition for another push. Go back and forth.

PERFORMANCE–Continuously for 30-60 seconds.

BREATHING–Inhale on the downward motion, exhale coming up.

variation

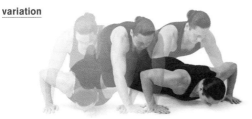

START POSITION–Push-up position with knees bent together (keep knees in the same position).

MOVEMENT–Perform a push-up with the knees bent, then bring hands together.

9. SHOULDER LATERAL LIFTS WITH SIDE SQUATS
(30–60 seconds)

Stand with dumbbells held at the side of the body. Stepping the right leg to the side, execute a squat while doing a shoulder lateral lift. Bring the right leg back to the beginning and repeat on the left side. Arms go up and knees bend at the same time.

Feet 1½ shoulder width across.

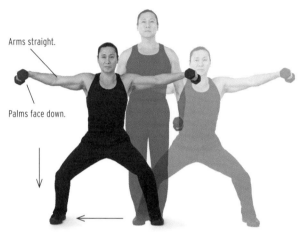

Arms straight.

Palms face down.

START POSITION–Stand tall, arms straight by your sides with palms facing body.

MOVEMENT–Move right foot sideways 1½ shoulder widths into a squat position while executing a shoulder lateral lift (hold slightly when arms are up), bring foot back and then repeat on the other side.

PERFORMANCE–Continuously for 30-60 seconds.

BREATHING–Inhale while arms are up and legs are bent.

10. REVERSE BACK ROWS (with straight leg heel kicks)
(30–60 seconds)

From the back row position, pull the arms into the chest, while lifting one leg straight to the rear, pushing the heel upward and pointing toes downward (hold). Repeat the same motion with the other leg. Try to keep the lifting leg as straight as possible.

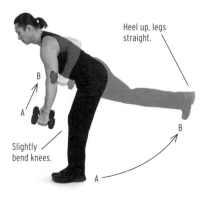

Heel up, legs straight.

B

A

Slightly bend knees.

B

A

START POSITION–Feet together, arms straight down from the body with palms facing each other.

MOVEMENT–Perform a reverse back row while executing a backward straight leg kick with the heel facing up holding at the top before switching legs.

PERFORMANCE–Alternate legs, performing continuously for 30-60 seconds.

BREATHING–Inhale when elbows and leg are up.

11. BICEP CURLS WITH FORWARD LUNGE

(30–60 seconds)

Standing straight with dumbbells next to the body, execute a right leg front lunge while simultaneously doing a bicep curl. Come back to original position and repeat on the other leg.

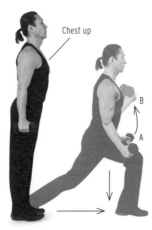

Chest up

11

B

A

START POSITION–Stand tall, arms extended by your sides with palms facing body.

MOVEMENT–Step forward into a front lunge, at the same time executing a bicep curl with both arms, then bring the foot back and repeat on the other side.

PERFORMANCE–Alternate legs, perform continuously for 30-60 seconds.

BREATHING–Inhale at the top of the bicep curl.

12. TRICEP KICKBACKS WITH REAR LEG CURLS

(30–60 seconds)

Perform a tricep kickback, while executing a rear leg curl with one leg. Repeat the movement with the other leg. Pull the leg up at the same time the arms extend backward.

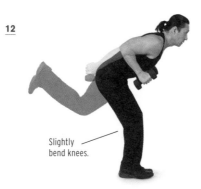

12

Slightly bend knees.

START POSITION–Bend body, keeping core region tight, feet together, elbows bent and tucked with arms next to the body.

MOVEMENT–Execute a tricep kick-back with both arms while performing a rear leg curl with one leg, then repeat with the other leg. Make sure to have the lifting leg at the highest point when both arms are extended back.

PERFORMANCE–Alternate legs, perform continuously for 30-60 seconds.

BREATHING–Inhale when arms are extended back and leg is lifted.

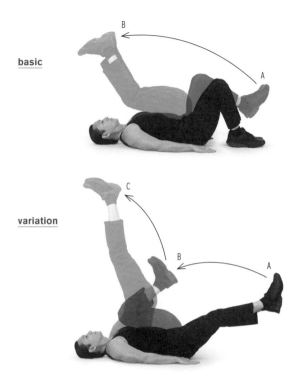

13. TWO MOTION STRAIGHT LEG LIFTS (30–60 seconds)
    Lying back with legs straight, hands flat and down the side of the
    body, lift the legs off the floor and point your toes. When your
    foot is pointing up, lift your hips and lower back off the floor.
    Then lower your body, extending the legs downward without
    touching the floor.

Stretching Plan Week 5: Brown Belt Advanced Level

Stretching goals:
1. Include all standing foundation stretches, and two entire body combination stretching routines. (Alternating arm rotations and full
   body rotations)
2. Perform standing bent leg and straight leg routines.
3. Learn side position Taekwondo stretching kicks, which will emphasize lower body and hip rotation.
4. Focus on floor stretches for the core/hip area to help develop greater
   lateral movement for the legs and body.

5. This level is all about cardio stretching, with continuous arm and leg routines. These exercises will help you develop better balance, coordination, and concentration.
6. Practice at least three days this week.

1. **STANDING FOUNDATION STRETCHES** (white/yellow level)
   1. Neck stretches

NECK LIFTS

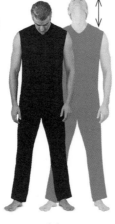

NECK TILTS

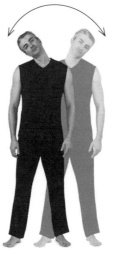

1.1a

1.1b

Your forehead-to-chin axis should be vertical.

NECK TURNS

NECK ROTATIONS

1.1c

1.1d

2. Shoulder stretches

UP / DOWN SHRUGS

Hold and squeeze at
the highest point for
two seconds.

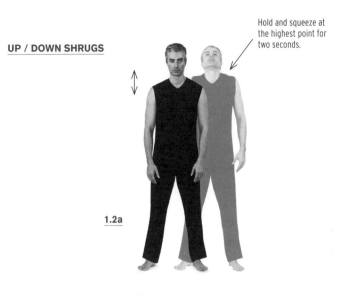

1.2a

FRONT / BACK SHRUGS

SHOULDER ROTATIONS

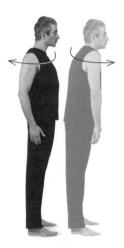

1.2b

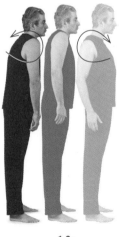

1.2c

3. Arm stretches

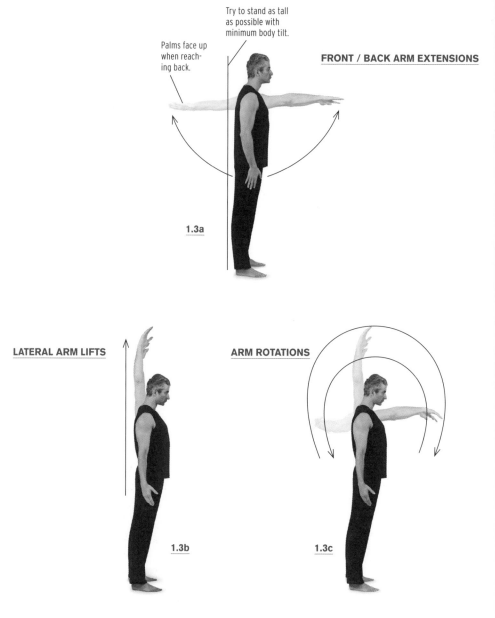

Try to stand as tall as possible with minimum body tilt.

Palms face up when reaching back.

FRONT / BACK ARM EXTENSIONS

1.3a

LATERAL ARM LIFTS

1.3b

ARM ROTATIONS

1.3c

4. Hip/pelvis stretches

FRONT / BACK PELVIC TILTS

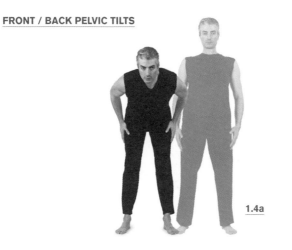

1.4a

SIDE-TO-SIDE PELVIC TILTS

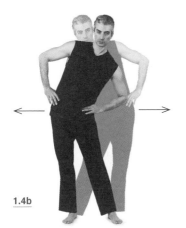

1.4b

HIP ROTATIONS

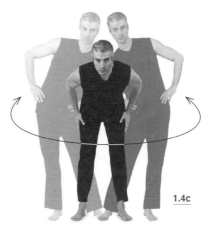

1.4c

5. Front and back leg combo stretches (hamstrings, calves, and groin muscles)

GROIN MUSCLE STRETCH

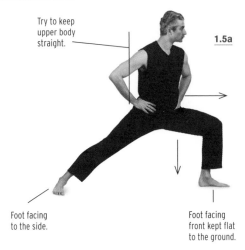

Try to keep upper body straight.

1.5a

Foot facing to the side.

Foot facing front kept flat to the ground.

HAMSTRING AND CALF STRETCH

1.5b

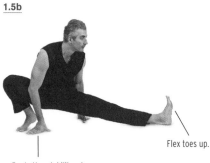

Flex toes up.

For better stability, place hands on the floor.

FRONT AND BACK LEG COMBO STRETCH

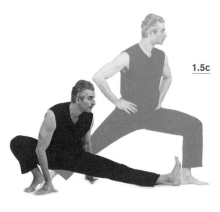

1.5c

6. Full body stretch

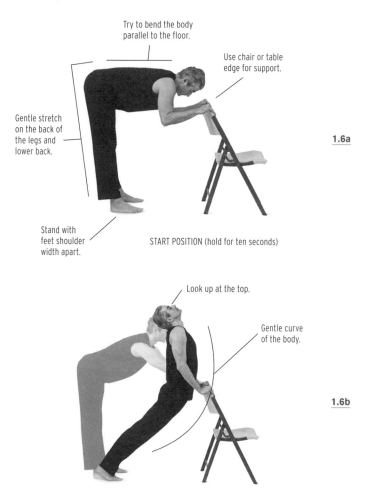

Try to bend the body parallel to the floor.

Use chair or table edge for support.

Gentle stretch on the back of the legs and lower back.

1.6a

Stand with feet shoulder width apart.

START POSITION (hold for ten seconds)

Look up at the top.

Gentle curve of the body.

1.6b

2. ALTERNATING ARM EXTENSIONS (green/blue level—arms, upper body, hamstrings)

This is a combined routine. First do individual arm extension moves A–D (eight times each). Then combine them in a routine starting with eight reps at each position, then six reps, then four reps, then two reps. Finally, at two reps at each position, repeat for eight sets.

Start Position—Stand upright with feet 1½ shoulder widths apart and arms straight.

Breathing—Exhale when reaching with arms.

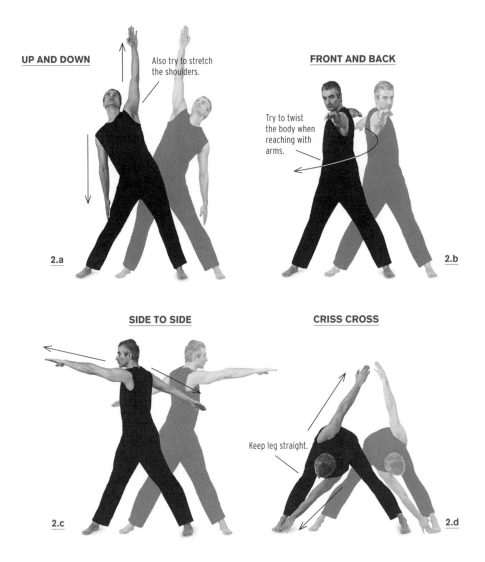

UP AND DOWN

Also try to stretch the shoulders.

2.a

FRONT AND BACK

Try to twist the body when reaching with arms.

2.b

SIDE TO SIDE

2.c

CRISS CROSS

Keep leg straight.

2.d

3. FULL BODY ROTATIONS
   (arms, upper body, and hamstrings)
   Start Position—Stand with legs two shoulder widths apart, keeping hands extended.
   Breathing—Exhale when stretching.
   A. DOWN AND UP—Keeping arms extended and holding hands together, reach downward toward the floor (hold). Straighten up and arch the body slightly backward, extending arms

upward. Repeat movement four times. Keep legs straight.

B. SIDE TO SIDE—Holding hands together, turn the body to the left side with your stomach facing down and extend the arms parallel to the floor. Then perform the stretch to the right side. Go back and forth four times. Feet should be two shoulder widths apart.

C. BODY ROTATION—Now combine all elements as if your body was a wheel. First reach to the floor, then turn to the left, keeping your body bent and arms extended; then circle back and up to the top, arching your body and extending arms upward; now reach to the right side, and finally back to the floor position. Perform rotation in the opposite direction. Repeat four times. (Do this stretch in a slow and smooth manner, inhaling halfway going up, and exhaling as you move down).

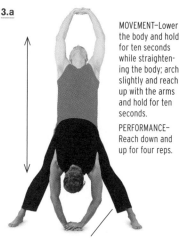

3.a

MOVEMENT–Lower the body and hold for ten seconds while straightening the body; arch slightly and reach up with the arms and hold for ten seconds.

PERFORMANCE–Reach down and up for four reps.

Keep legs straight.

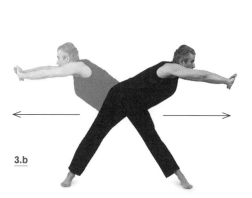

3.b

MOVEMENT–While bending, turn the body to one side with arms extended (hold for ten seconds). Repeat on the other side.

PERFORMANCE–Go from one side to the other four times.

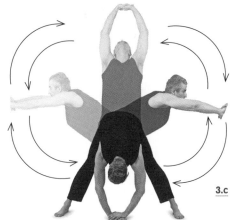

3.c

MOVEMENT–Starting from the down position, complete a full-body circle with both arms extended, going in one direction. Then repeat in the other direction. Alternate from one side to the other.

PERFORMANCE–Perform in a smooth manner, inhaling going up and exhaling coming down, for four reps.

4. ALTERNATING KNEE KICKS (core and hips)
Start Position—Stand tall and alternate bringing one knee up and then the other.

Breathing—Gently exhale when lifting the leg.

A. STRAIGHT UP KNEE KICK—
Bring the left knee straight up,
followed by the right knee. Repeat
eight times.

B. OPPOSITE SHOULDER KNEE
KICK—Cross the left knee to the
right side of the body while bringing arms to the left side, then
bring the right knee to left side
while arms swing to the right.
Repeat eight times.

C. SAME SHOULDER KNEE KICK—
Bring the left knee to the outside
of the left shoulder while stretching arms downward, then do
the same with right leg. Repeat eight times.

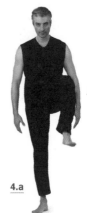

MOVEMENT–Alternate by bringing one knee straight up and then the other.

PERFORMANCE–Alternate legs for a total of eight reps.

4.a

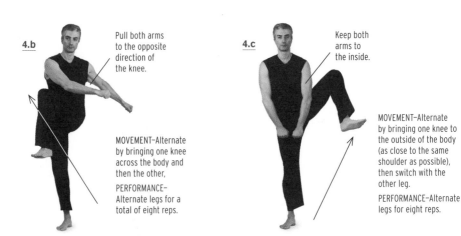

4.b

Pull both arms to the opposite direction of the knee.

MOVEMENT–Alternate by bringing one knee across the body and then the other,

PERFORMANCE–Alternate legs for a total of eight reps.

4.c

Keep both arms to the inside.

MOVEMENT–Alternate by bringing one knee to the outside of the body (as close to the same shoulder as possible), then switch with the other leg.

PERFORMANCE–Alternate legs for eight reps.

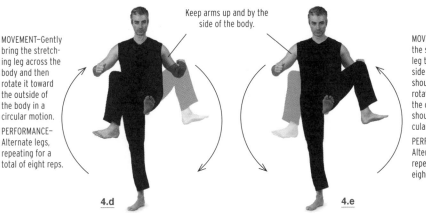

Keep arms up and by the side of the body.

MOVEMENT–Gently bring the stretching leg across the body and then rotate it toward the outside of the body in a circular motion.

PERFORMANCE–Alternate legs, repeating for a total of eight reps.

MOVEMENT–Bring the stretching leg toward the side of the same shoulder, the rotate it toward the opposite shoulder in a circular motion.

PERFORMANCE–Alternate legs, repeating for eight reps.

4.d   **4.e**

D. OUTSIDE CIRCULAR KNEE KICK—Execute an outward circular knee kick with the left leg while keeping arms up. Do the same with the right leg. Repeat eight times.

E. INSIDE CIRCULAR KNEE KICK—Execute an inward circular kick with the left knee, keeping the arms up. Do the same with the right knee. Repeat eight times.

5. ALTERNATING STRAIGHT LEG KICKS (core, hips, and legs)
These are the same moves as the alternating knee kicks, but keep the legs straight.

Start Position—Start upright with both feet almost touching each other, and make sure to limit any excess movement of the upper body when stretching.

Breathing—exhale when lifting the legs.

A. STRAIGHT LEG FRONT KICK—Bring the left leg up and down in a straight position without tilting the body, then with other leg. Repeat eight times.

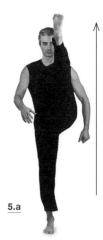

MOVEMENT–Bring stretching leg straight up, then switch to other leg.

PERFORMANCE–Alternate stretching legs for a total of eight reps.

5.a

B. OPPOSITE SHOULDER STRAIGHT LEG KICK—Lift left leg diagonally across the body to the right side and back down, then do the same with other leg. Repeat eight times.

C. SAME SHOULDER STRAIGHT LEG KICK—Lift left leg diagonally to the outside of the body while keeping both arms centered, then do the same with other leg. Repeat eight times.

D. OUTSIDE CIRCULAR STRAIGHT LEG KICK—Execute an outside circular stretch with the left leg, then do the same with other leg. Repeat eight times.

E. INSIDE CIRCULAR STRAIGHT LEG KICK—Execute a inside circular stretch with the left leg while keeping arms raised, then do the same with other leg. Repeat eight times.

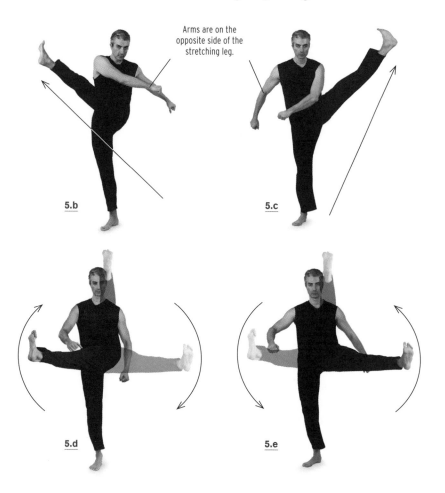

Arms are on the opposite side of the stretching leg.

5.b

5.c

5.d

5.e

6. SIDE POSITION STRAIGHT LEG STRETCHES WITH CHAIR
(legs and hips)
Start Position—Stand upright while holding the chair at the highest point, at arm's distance, with the same support hand and leg
closest to the chair. Point the support foot toward the chair and
position sideways, making sure to lean back sideways when lifting
the stretching leg.

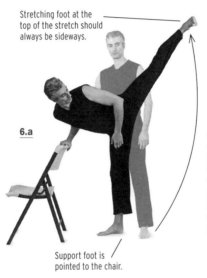

Stretching foot at the
top of the stretch should
always be sideways.

6.a

MOVEMENT—Lean back side-
ways, lowering the body
toward the chair while lifting
the other straight leg up in a
side position.

PERFORMANCE—Perform four
reps on one leg in a slow and
controlled manner, then repeat on the other leg.

Support foot is
pointed to the chair.

A. SIDE STRETCH KICK—Stand with the right supporting foot
   pointed to the back part of the chair, while the left foot is
   turned sideways (perpendicular to the right foot). Your body
   should be in line with the supporting foot. While lifting the
   left leg up, tilt your body sideways toward the supporting hand
   and right leg. Repeat four times, then go to other leg.
B. HOOK STRETCH KCK—Stand the same way as the side
   stretch, but as you're leaning sideways lift the stretching leg
   slightly to the front of your body, then gently swing the
   stretching leg backward in a circular manner, leading with
   your heel. Pretend your leg is going over an object. Try to keep
   your toes the same height as the heel while keeping the leg as
   horizontal as possible. Repeat four times, then go to other leg.
   Keep the toes and heel the same height.

C. ROUNDHOUSE STRETCH KICK—Stand the same way as in the previous stretches, but change the feet positions. Place your support foot position where it points to about a 45 degree angle to the support chair. As you're leaning back toward the chair, rotate the left leg in a circular motion, toward the front of your body leading with the toes (opposite rotation of the hook stretch kick). Repeat four times, then go to other leg.

6.b

Keep foot sideways.

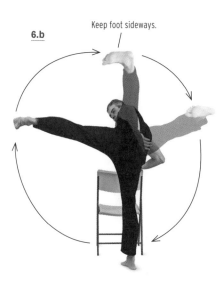

6.c

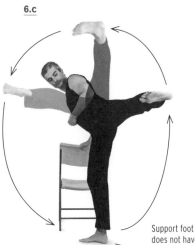

Support foot does not have to be fully pointed toward the chair.

MOVEMENT–While leaning sideways, first lift the stretching leg toward the front of the body, then gently circle the leg up and backward (lead with the heel part of the foot).

PERFORMANCE–Perform four reps in a circular motion on one leg and then repeat on the other.

MOVEMENT–Lean sideways while lifting the stretching leg slightly behind the body, then gently circle the leg forward, leading with the toes (opposite rotation of the hook stretch).

PERFORMANCE–Repeat four times on each leg.

7. SEATED FOUNDATION FLOOR STRETCHES
(hamstrings, calves, groin muscles, hips, lower back)

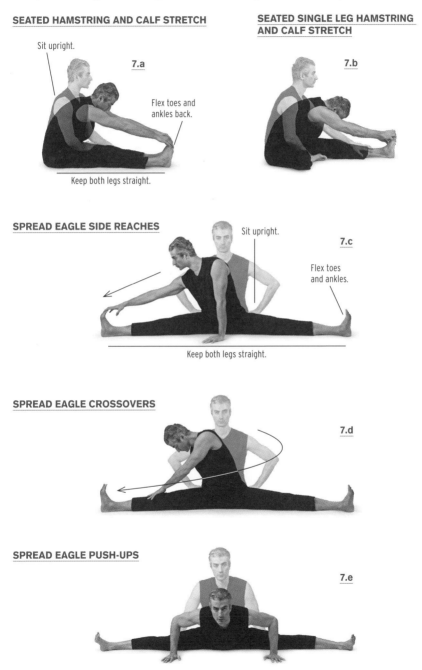

SEATED HAMSTRING AND CALF STRETCH

Sit upright.

7.a

Flex toes and ankles back.

Keep both legs straight.

SEATED SINGLE LEG HAMSTRING AND CALF STRETCH

7.b

SPREAD EAGLE SIDE REACHES

Sit upright.

7.c

Flex toes and ankles.

Keep both legs straight.

SPREAD EAGLE CROSSOVERS

7.d

SPREAD EAGLE PUSH-UPS

7.e

8. LYING BACK FOUNDATION FLOOR STRETCHES
(core, lower back, hips)

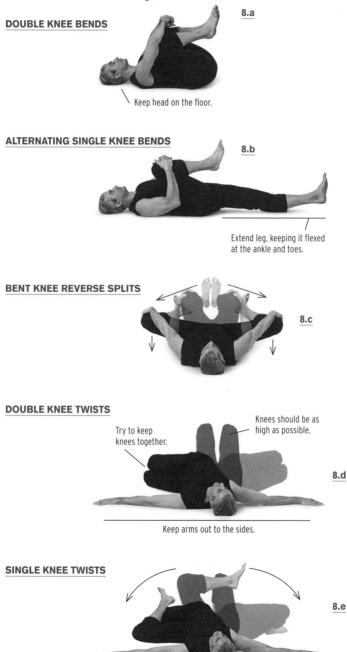

DOUBLE KNEE BENDS

8.a

Keep head on the floor.

ALTERNATING SINGLE KNEE BENDS

8.b

Extend leg, keeping it flexed at the ankle and toes.

BENT KNEE REVERSE SPLITS

8.c

DOUBLE KNEE TWISTS

Try to keep knees together.

Knees should be as high as possible.

8.d

Keep arms out to the sides.

SINGLE KNEE TWISTS

8.e

9. LYING BACK STRAIGHT LEG STRETCHES (green/blue level)

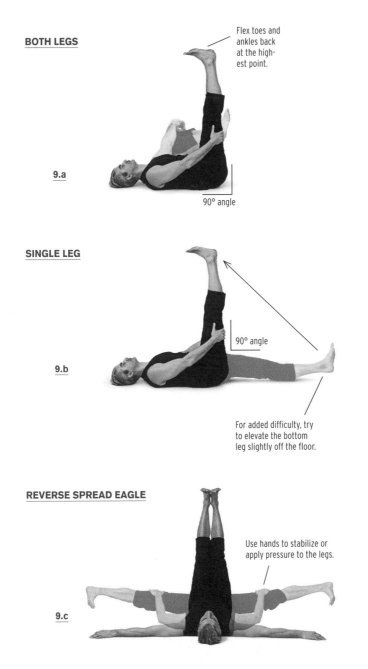

BOTH LEGS

Flex toes and ankles back at the highest point.

9.a

90° angle

SINGLE LEG

90° angle

9.b

For added difficulty, try to elevate the bottom leg slightly off the floor.

REVERSE SPREAD EAGLE

Use hands to stabilize or apply pressure to the legs.

9.c

WIPER BLADE STRETCH

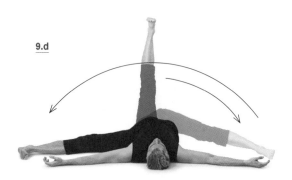

9.d

10. FLOOR FACING STRETCHES (lower back and groin muscles)
Start Position—On the floor in a kneeling position.
Breathing—Exhale when applying pressure downward.

   A. BENT KNEE SIDE SPLIT—Go onto your hands and knees and spread your knees as far as you can. Then gently sway your pelvic area forward and backward four times. Try to hold at the lowest point for at least 10 seconds.

Keep body facing front.

10.a

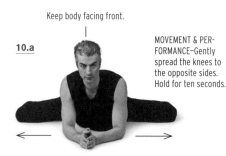

MOVEMENT & PERFORMANCE—Gently spread the knees to the opposite sides. Hold for ten seconds.

   B. SINGLE LEG SIDE SPLIT—From a kneeling position, keep your right knee bent while extending the left leg out to the side, sliding the inside of the foot and straightening the leg along the floor. (You should make a straight line from the bended knee through the pelvic region to the heel part of the left foot.) When you can't extend any farther, sway your upper

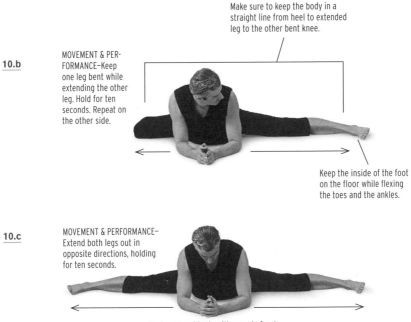

10.b MOVEMENT & PER-
FORMANCE—Keep
one leg bent while
extending the other
leg. Hold for ten
seconds. Repeat on
the other side.

Make sure to keep the body in a
straight line from heel to extended
leg to the other bent knee.

Keep the inside of the foot
on the floor while flexing
the toes and the ankles.

10.c MOVEMENT & PERFORMANCE—
Extend both legs out in
opposite directions, holding
for ten seconds.

Try to support body with arms in front.

body forward and backward. Repeat on the other leg. Try to
hold at the lowest point for at least 10 seconds.

Keep the inside of your foot on the floor while flexing toes
and ankles

C. FULL SIDE SPLIT—Keeping your legs straight while supporting your body with both arms, extend both legs outward (hold
for at least 10 seconds).

Eating Plan Week 5: Brown Belt Advanced Level

Drink a minimum of eight glasses of water per day as per previous instructions.

This week, to help your body adjust to the new food portions, your
meal consumption will stay the same as week 4.

Your meals are now the new reduced portions, except for breakfast—that means three meals and two healthy snacks per day.

RED BELT ADVANCED LEVEL (WEEK SIX)– GOAL WITHIN REACH/DON'T GIVE UP!

This is a stage where I've seen a lot of people drop out. Impossible, you say! Not really, some people feel as if they know and have done it all by this time. Unfortunately, this is a bit premature. It's as if one feels that high school is sufficient, and that there is no need to go to college.

That's why we signify this level as red, a level of danger or a false level of confidence or security.

I'm sure most of you have seen the film *Star Wars* and remember who Darth Vader is. Besides being the bad guy, he was the one that did not have the patience and understanding that was needed to make him complete. Instead, he let conceit dominate his actions and became evil. This concept, used in *Star Wars*, is obviously from the teachings of the martial arts. From the thousands of black belts that I've awarded in my lifetime I can tell you that double, maybe even triple, that number of students stopped at this red belt stage.

Strengthening Plan Week 6: Red Belt Advanced Level

Strength goals:
1. Perform all the fundamental calisthenics for 45–60 seconds each.
2. Perform all the previous dumbbell exercises for 45–60 seconds.
3. Perform all the combined dumbbell and leg exercises for 45–60 seconds.
4. Continue from one exercise to the next without rest.
5. Perform three days this week.

    1. PUSH-UPS (45–60 seconds)
    2. LEG SQUATS (45–60 seconds)
    3. LYING BACK BENT LEG LIFTS (45–60 seconds)
    4. REVERSE BACK ROWS (45–60 seconds)
    5. SHOULDER LATERAL LIFTS (45–60 seconds)
    6. TRICEP KICKBACKS (45–60 seconds)
    7. BICEP CURLS (45–60 seconds)
    8. LATERAL PUSH-UPS (45–60 seconds)

9. SHOULDER LATERAL LIFTS WITH SIDE SQUATS
   (45–60 seconds)
10. REVERSE BACK ROWS with straight leg heel kicks
    (45–60 seconds)
11. BICEP CURLS WITH FORWARD LUNGE (45–60 seconds)
12. TRICEP KICKBACKS WITH REAR LEG CURLS
    (45–60 seconds)
13. TWO MOTION STRAIGHT LEG LIFTS (45–60 seconds)

Stretching Plan Week 6: Red Belt Advanced Level

Stretching goals:
1. Continue with the same exercises from the previous level, while pacing your routines properly for a full cardio workout.
2. Perform a minimum of three days this week.

Eating Plan Week 6: Red Belt Advanced Level

Continue with the water, of course, but by now soft drinks and juice should really be out of the picture.

Continue with the same breakfast and lunch consumption as week 5. Your body should be adjusting to the new portions. But now I want you to reduce the new dinner portion by a quarter.

Now breakfast is the biggest meal of the day, lunch the second biggest, and dinner the smallest.

You should now be eating three healthy meals and two healthy snacks.

Michael's Thoughts on Being an Advanced Belt

An interesting thing that happens when you start to exercise is that your desire to be healthy starts to kick in. Which means instead of forcing yourself to eat healthy, you're just going to want to eat healthy. Because you're starting to feel good, you're starting to breathe better. You'll want to quit smoking. You'll want to not order that second bottle of wine when you go out to dinner. You'll want to not wake up with that hangover. You'll start to find you'll go out to dinner and it'll be easier to make a healthy choice, because you just feel better.

Also, mental clarity improves. When you work out in Taekwondo, you can't think of anything else. I don't care what you're going through in your day, you might be facing bankruptcy, you might be signing a mortgage, you might be under a lot of stress because business is going really bad. Once you start working out, you can't think of any of that stuff, because it takes all your focus and concentration to execute the techniques. It's not like the gym, where you're watching CNN or listening to music or books on tape, so you're working out but thinking about something else. It's impossible to do that in Taekwondo. So your mind is completely engaged. And when you train like that regularly, without a doubt you're going to see an increase in your mental focus and clarity.

I think it also helps with managing stress. We all have a lot of stress. Living in New York City, you have to deal with stress on a constant basis. It kind of helps you open up a space in your mind to deal with stress. You'll find yourself becoming a little bit more patient.

Over 10 years of training, I've met many other martial artists, and talking with them, I've noticed a lot of them have said they felt like they've reached a plateau around the advanced belt mark. I never felt I reached a place where I couldn't improve. All I had to do was look at students and instructors who were higher belts and more proficient than me. That always gives me inspiration, especially watching the instructors. When you watch martial arts being done by someone who's a master, you really see the art of it. There's a beauty in the movements. There's fluidity and a balance and power. If you watch Grandmaster do forms, that's art in motion. It gives you something to aspire to. I always got a lot of inspiration from watching that. I always felt I wanted to keep going. Training with Grandmaster, quitting never entered my mind. There were times when I had to leave town—I lived in Detroit for a year and I would come back on the weekends. I would always try to make a class, even if it was only once or twice a month. But the idea of quitting never, ever entered my mind.

BLACK BELT ADVANCED LEVEL (WEEK SEVEN AND BEYOND)—CONFIDENCE AND MATURITY

Congratulations! You've made it!

By achieving this level, you've proven that you're serious about taking charge of your life and that you've prioritized fitness and nutrition into your daily routine.

Unless you've trained in the martial arts, people don't quite understand the meaning of a black belt. Let me give you a martial arts definition of what a black belt signifies:

The color black signifies knowledge or maturity. It's a level of a new beginning, where you understand the fundamentals. You've learned how to be patient, and how important patience is if you want to continue the learning process. You've learned to be humble and to stay focused and persevere, no matter what external factors come your way. And the main thing that makes a black belt special is how it makes you feel inside. Don't compare yourself with others. Instead, be the best that you can be.

How can you apply this principle in life?

Too often in our lives, we give up before even making an attempt or think that we know the conclusion of something without knowing the story. Life is what you make it to be—utilize that new confidence and take charge of it. Don't let another day go by in boredom, keep it exciting, have a positive attitude. Remember the excitement you felt when you were going on that special trip, where getting there was half the fun. Keep that attitude for the rest of your life and make now the beginning of the journey, not the end.

Strengthening Plan Week 7 and Beyond: Black Belt Advanced Level

Strength goals:
1. Perform all the exercises from the red belt level for 60 seconds each.
2. Do not take any rest in-between exercises.
3. If you have time, try to repeat the entire sequence of exercises again, or parts of the sequence at least one or two days out of three.
4. Always do these exercises three days per week.

Stretching goals:

1. Perform standing foundation exercises everyday.
2. Do appropriate stretches to get you warmed up.
3. Perform the black belt stretching form five times.
4. Perform all the floor stretches from all the levels together as a routine.
5. Stretching is lubrication to the body, so frequency is vital to keep your body from injuries.

Black Belt Stretching Form

This stretching form is a culmination of all the previous stretching exercises that you've been doing for the past six weeks. One of the reasons for creating this stretching form is because I believe individual stretches are good, but I feel they are not adequate to get the entire body moving and warmed up. This is a form that I've created that loosens and warms up all the muscles and joints, from head to toe. For a video demonstration, please visit my website at www.tkangtkd.com.

BLACK BELT STRETCHING FORM (40 continuous movements)
Start position—stand upright with legs approximately shoulder-width apart.

1. **Neck Rotations**
   Complete a full circle with the neck, inhaling as you rotate up, exhaling on the downward movement. Repeat four times.

   A. Rotate starting left.
   B. Rotate starting right.
   C. Repeat steps 1 and 2.

   BREATHING– inhale going up, exhale going down.

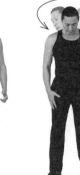
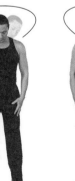
Rotate neck to the left.
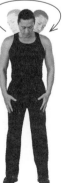
Rotate neck to the right.

2. **Stationary Arm Rotations**

Complete a full circle with both arms, inhaling upward and exhaling downward. Repeat four times.

A. Rotate both arms backward.

B. Rotate both arms forward.

C. Repeat steps A and B.

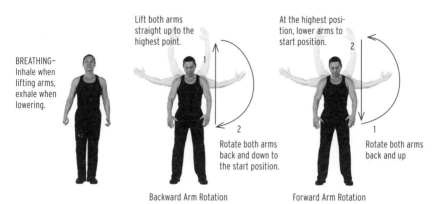

BREATHING–
Inhale when lifting arms, exhale when lowering.

Lift both arms straight up to the highest point.

Rotate both arms back and down to the start position.

Backward Arm Rotation

At the highest position, lower arms to start position.

Rotate both arms back and up

Forward Arm Rotation

3. **Arm Rotations with Front and Back Lunge**

Do one side twice, then repeat on the other side. Repeat exercise four times.

A. Extending both arms forward, step to the front with the left leg into a deep lunge position, then gently rotate both arms backward, completing a full circle, stopping arms at the original extended position (inhale during this move). Then step back with the left leg into a right leg lunge position while completing a full circle forward rotation with both arms, ending with arms extended back with palms facing up (exhale during this move).

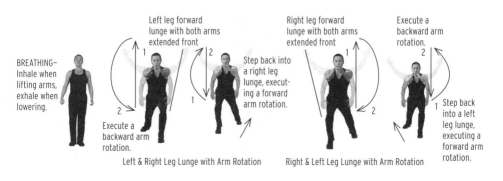

BREATHING–
Inhale when lifting arms, exhale when lowering.

Left leg forward lunge with both arms extended front

Execute a backward arm rotation.

Step back into a right leg lunge, executing a forward arm rotation.

Left & Right Leg Lunge with Arm Rotation

Right leg forward lunge with both arms extended front

Execute a backward arm rotation.

Step back into a left leg lunge, executing a forward arm rotation.

Right & Left Leg Lunge with Arm Rotation

B. Repeat the sequence on the same side.

C. Extending both arms forward, step to the front with the right leg into a deep lunge position, then gently rotate both arms backward, completing a full circle, stopping arms at the original extended position (inhale during this move). Then step back with right leg into a left leg lunge position while completing a full circle forward rotation with both arms, ending with arms extended back with palms facing up (exhale during this move).

D. Repeat the sequence on the same side.

4. **Sideways Extensions**

   Exhale when extending arms. Repeat movement four times.

   A. Looking left, step left leg out to the side more than shoulder width into a low squat position, while extending arms out to each side.

   B. Bring left foot back and repeat on right side.

   C. Repeat on left side.

   D. Repeat on right side.

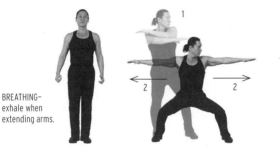 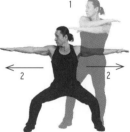

BREATHING—exhale when extending arms.

Move left into a saddle stance while extending arms to opposite sides.

Move right into a saddle stance while extending arms to opposite sides.

5. **Sideways Arm Circles**

   Exhale during circular arm movement. Repeat four times.

   A. Turn sideways stepping with the left leg into a deep front lunge position while rotating both arms in a circle, as if you were turning a big steering wheel.

   B. Bring the left foot back to the starting point and repeat the exercise, stepping with the right leg.

C. Repeat to the left.

D. Repeat to the right.

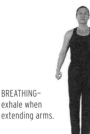 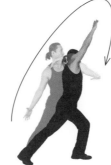 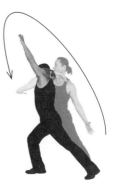

BREATHING—
exhale when
extending arms.

Turn left into a left leg lunge,
rotating both arms to the left,
as if you are turning a big wheel.

Turn right into a right leg lunge,
rotating both arms to the right.

6. **Alternating Knee Kicks**

   Standing on the spot, exhale when lifting knee. Repeat four times.

   A. Bring left knee up.

   B. Bring right knee up.

   C. Bring left knee up.

   D. Bring right knee up.

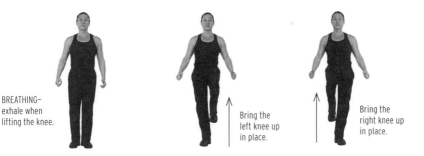

BREATHING—
exhale when
lifting the knee.

Bring the
left knee up
in place.

Bring the
right knee up
in place.

7. **Circular Outside and Inside Combination Knee Kicks**

   Exhale when lifting knee. Repeat four times.

   A. Turn left, executing a left leg circular outside knee kick,
      followed by a right leg circular inside knee kick combination.

   B. Turn right, executing a right leg circular outside knee kick,
      followed by a left leg circular inside knee kick combination.

C. Repeat to the left side.

D. Repeat to right side.

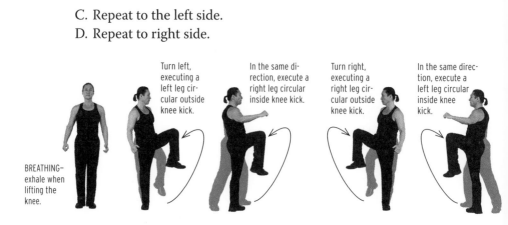

BREATHING—exhale when lifting the knee.

8. **Circular Outside and Inside Combination Straight Leg Kicks**
   Exhale when lifting legs. Repeat four times.

   A. Turn left, executing a left leg circular outside straight leg kick, followed by a right leg circular inside straight leg kick combination.

   B. Turn right, executing a right leg circular outside straight leg kick, followed by a left leg circular inside straight leg kick combination.

BREATHING—exhale when kicking

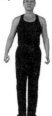
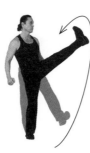
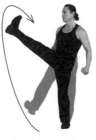
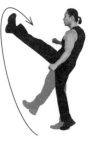

Turn left, executing a left leg circular outside straight leg kick.

In the same direction, execute a right leg circular inside straight leg kick.

Turn right, executing a right leg circular outside straight leg kick.

In the same direction, execute a left leg circular inside straight leg kick.

C. Repeat to left side.

D. Repeat to right side.

9. **Front and Side Combination Straight Leg Kicks**
   Exhale when lifting legs. Repeat four times.
   A. Execute a left leg straight kick to the front, lower, then execute a left leg straight side kick to the back.
   B. Execute a right leg straight kick to the front, lower, then execute a right leg straight side kick to the back.
   C. Repeat with the left leg.
   D. Repeat with the right leg.

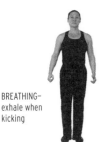 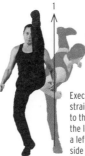 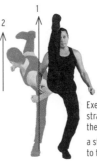

BREATHING– exhale when kicking

Execute a left leg straight leg front kick to the front, then lower the leg and execute a left leg straight leg side kick to the back.

Execute a right leg straight leg front kick to the front, followed by a straight leg side kick to the back.

10. **Hook and Roundhouse Combination Straight Leg Kicks**
    Exhale when lifting legs. Repeat four times.
    A. Execute a left leg straight hook stretch kick to the back, lower, then execute a left leg straight roundhouse kick to the left side.
    B. Execute a right leg straight hook stretch kick to the back, lower, then execute a right leg straight roundhouse stretch kick to the right side.
    C. Repeat with the left leg.
    D. Repeat with the right leg.

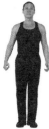 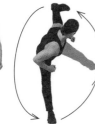 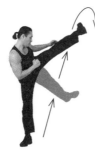 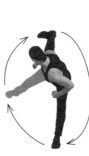

BREATHING– exhale when kicking.

Execute a left leg straight leg hook kick to the back.

Lower the leg, then execute a left leg straight leg roundhouse kick to the left side.

Execute a right leg straight leg hook kick to the back.

Lower the leg, then execute a right leg straight leg roundhouse kick to the right side.

FORMS FOR MEDITATION

Most individuals have very little understanding of what meditation is. They often visualize it as sitting with your legs folded, eyes closed, arms and hands in certain gesture positions, accompanied by calm, slow breathing.

In traditional martial arts we practice and perform forms or patterns. Think of it like imaginary fighting, or shadow boxing. If you've ever seen people doing Tai Chi, what do you think they're doing? Does it look like dance, or some kind of slow-moving ballet? Apparently, they are mimicking the movements of a fight—they are in an imaginary battle scenario against multiple opponents. You're probably thinking, how come they're doing it so slowly? The thing about forms is that depending on the different styles of martial arts, it can vary in speed, power, and intensity. Also, it is very common that even in the same discipline, there are many different types of forms—slow and fast, or soft and hard. As a matter of fact, more advanced forms sometimes have a combination of all these elements.

Often, people not familiar with martial arts question how these forms can be useful in a real confrontation: "I just want to learn to fight or defend myself, I've got no time for this nonsense."

What people don't understand is that the main thing you learn by practicing forms is meditation, and concentration. You're probably surprised at this.

In martial arts, things such as hitting a bag, breaking bricks/boards, and fighting are all exercises in meditation, but in many ways a lot easier than doing forms. I'm sure you're wondering how that is possible. Well, if you carefully assess the other scenarios, there already exists a predetermined goal. For example, if you're breaking an object, obviously your goal has been established by the type of object. If you're fighting, what else is there to do than fight and try to beat your opponent?

But when you're doing a form, what is your goal? You're not hitting an object or fighting anyone, there's nothing or no one you have to compete against.

But that's what makes doing forms so difficult, because you're on stage all alone—basically, it's a one person show. If you make a mistake or lose your balance or your hand or body posture is not correct, it's going to show. Not like a fight situation, where you can get lucky or your opponent can make a mistake and you can take advantage of it. Also when doing forms, you have to be able to psyche yourself up without the help of external forces. What I mean by external forces are when there's a few boards in front of you to break, those boards give you an immediate goal or challenge. Or your opponent attacking you during a match—you're forced to fight back.

When doing forms, you have to know precisely when to turn that energy on or off, and at the same time your memory of the sequence and moves has to be perfect. To me, performing forms is meditation at its highest level, since your body and mind have to become one. Think about it, while you're in motion you have to be focused—that's why I call it "Meditation in Motion." The traditional sitting down and meditating exercises are very passive compared to doing something like this.

Why is this such a great exercise? Well, think about it: in busy modern life, where we are constantly trying to remember so many things, this type of exercise will train our bodies and minds to stay focused, even under the most stressful circumstances.

Think about when a child is given a reading assignment, and their biggest problem is concentration. It doesn't matter if you assign them a chapter, or even a page for that matter, if their brain doesn't have that ability to focus and memorize, nothing's going in. I feel that there should be required courses that teachers must take, where they are taught concentration exercises that they can do in the classroom with the kids. I can tell you from my experience in teaching martial arts to kids, practicing forms is the number one way to develop greater focus.

I can also tell you that if you do traditional meditation exercises with the kids it will never work. Why? How are you going to get this active child to remain still? Again, that's why I emphasize forms training. It gives them a task, a goal, while also training their memory. The other super important ingredient is that it develops patience. Patience is the key element in developing focus.

In martial arts training, we often practice the same form for months, sometimes even years. It sounds boring! Not at all: each time we do it, we try to fine-tune it and make improvements. Maybe the first time we'll do it fast, then slow; we might emphasize deeper stances; execute higher kicks; or stronger hand motions, better balance, and so on. By practicing the same element over and over, perfection being the ultimate goal, you develop patience; and in return, this becomes an exercise in meditation.

Even though some of the exercise routines might feel repetitious, you have to stay focused. What you're trying to develop at this stage is muscle memory, both physical and mental stamina, and the only way that's going to happen is with repetition and some patience.

Eating for Week 7 and the Rest of Your Life

At this point, you're making smarter decisions about what you eat and drink. Think of food as fuel for your body. The more you can incorporate whole, non-processed food into your diet, the better your body will function. But if you get a craving for dessert or junk food, don't deny yourself.

If I eat a lot of the bad foods I know are not good for me, immediately the next day I will exercise harder than usual or cut down on the calories I eat, to get my body back in balance. The key is to not make it a habit by eating poorly or not exercising for many days.

You can still have your favorite foods, but eat them occasionally and in moderation.

Simple Eating Tips to Keep You Going

1. Drink lots of water.

    There's a reason I stress drinking water in my eating plan. Not only does it keep your body hydrated, which is a necessity (especially when working out), but it also flushes out toxins from your body. By drinking water throughout the day and especially before meals, it can also help you control hunger. If you feel hungry after a recent meal or snack, drinking water might be a solution, because your body may be in need of hydration rather than more food. Water intake is crucial for maintaining a balanced eating habit.

2. Eat what you are craving early in the day.

    If you're anything like me, food is one of your passions—I live for it. If I'm craving something fatty or salty or sweet, I try to eat it as part of the early meals during the day. This includes steak, ice cream, and even cake. Nothing is wrong with eating fats or sweets, as long as you do it in moderation. If you deprive yourself of the things you crave, you'll never stick with any eating regimen. We're trying to create a lifestyle that we can maintain, not a temporary eating plan.

3. Load up on vegetables and fruits.

Try to add servings of vegetables to all your meals. Vegetables are a great substitute for processed carbs. A salad along with lunch and dinner can also help you fill up. Eat lean proteins and low-fat dairy products along with vegetables. Fruits are a great way to replace any sugar craving. They make great snacks and also taste great chopped up in salads to add flavor.

4. Choose whole foods over processed foods.

Eating whole foods is imperative to staying healthy. Your body digests food better when it is closest to its natural state. When foods are too processed, not only can they lack nutritional value, but they can also be packed with sodium, trans fats, sugars, and preservatives. Certain small changes can make a big difference. For example, grilled chicken is a much better choice than highly processed chicken nuggets, and natural whole grains are a better choice than breads containing high-fructose corn syrup.

5. Snack in-between meals.

Eat snacks halfway between your main meals so you won't feel so hungry throughout the day. Snacking will keep your energy up and help you to not overeat at meal times. Replace oily, sugary, or salty snacks with foods like yogurt, fruit, veggies, or nuts. When I'm craving potato chips, I turn to nuts. Not only are they good for you, but they satisfy my craving for something salty and crunchy.

6. Use olive oil over other vegetable oils or animal fats.

Olive oil and seed oils are healthy alternatives to other cooking fats, which help lower bad cholesterol and increase good cholesterol. Not only is it better to cook with olive oil than butter, but it also adds flavor to foods like salads or roasted vegetables and meats.

7. Limit your intake of non-water beverages.
   Whether it's soft drinks, juices, or alcohol, be very aware that these drinks contain lots of sugar. These are filled with empty calories, so make sure to drink them sparingly. If you're craving juice, try to make your own homemade juice with a juicer. That way you know there are no artificial ingredients in the juice. If you don't have access to a juicer, mix juice with water if you want to drink something sweet.

8. Be aware of eating because of boredom or for emotional reasons.
   If you're not hungry, don't eat. Listen to your body. Often, we eat because we're bored or stressed and know a certain food will make us feel better. Instead of stocking your pantry with junk foods you know you will turn to if you're bored or unhappy, fill it with healthy alternatives. I'm sure you might have already heard this tip, but if you're not hungry enough to eat an apple, then you're probably not really hungry.

9. Read food labels.
   Products that claim to be "healthy" may be loaded with ingredients like high fructose corn syrup. I tell my students their safety is their own personal responsibility. It's the same with what you eat—it's your responsibility to read food labels and make sure your choices won't negatively impact a balanced eating habit.

10. Keep a positive attitude and be patient!
    Don't be discouraged if you can't see results right away! Your weight gain did not occur overnight, and neither will weight loss. It's a process that takes time—but be patient because it's not too late! Physical and mental changes will occur by following a simple nutrition and exercise plan that you can stick to in the long run.

Depending on your weight-loss goals, you can also try my pound a week plan that has worked very well for my students.

Aim to lose one pound a week. It may not sound like a lot, but keep it up for a year and you'll lose 50 pounds! Losing 50 pounds is a tremendous accomplishment! I believe losing 50 pounds over a year is a lot easier (and safer, and a lot more likely to actually happen) than trying to lose 50 pounds in one month and keeping the weight off for a year.

Usually people laugh when I tell them that their goal should be to lose just one pound a week if they're serious about losing weight and getting in shape. Yes, you're right; if you do something extreme, maybe you can lost 20 pounds in one month. But what happens in the second month, or the third (if you even get there)? Do you think you can continue at that pace? The truth is even if you can, you have a great chance of totally destroying your metabolism. Remember that a pound a week amounts to over 50 pounds in a year—that's a huge number!

The math is that 3500 calories equals one pound. So if you wanted to lose a pound a week, you have to somehow eliminate 3500 calories, or to break it down, 500 calories per day. That could mean perhaps one of your meals during the day has to be eliminated or reduced or that you'll have to spend approximately an hour or so working out at a pretty brisk pace on the treadmill, cycle or elliptical machine every day of the week. I think both options are pretty rough to do on a daily basis.

My approach is simple—give a little bit daily from each category. Reduce your food intake by 10%–15%, which can amount to 200–300 calories per day. You don't have to skip a meal, just eat a few bites less at each meal and eliminated calories will add up throughout the day. At the same time, try to burn off a similar amount of calories (200–300) per day through exercise, or by keeping more active (such as walking or biking to work if distance permits, taking stairs instead of elevators, or parking your car farther away when you go shopping). I think this method is achievable and a lot less stressful, especially when it needs to be done everyday.

I think it's easier for many people to become millionaires than to lose weight. Weight loss is one of the toughest challenges in life. Don't worry what other people are thinking. Remember that you're not alone!

Michael's Thoughts on Being a Black Belt

In Taekwondo, the good thing about the belt system is that it inspires you to keep pushing yourself. If you're doing the same old workout at the same old level and not trying to improve on your techniques or strength or stretching, you'll start to get bored. Which is why I probably never could stick to a gym. But getting a black belt is a big accomplishment. Getting one stripe or two stripes on your black belt, and learning a new form and new techniques is exciting. When you start and you're a white, yellow, or green belt and you see these black belts doing these forms, or you see one of the instructors when they take a class and they do 20-plus forms and they're dripping wet with sweat and you're like, "Oh my God!" it's inspiring and exciting! And 10 years later, you're doing 22 forms! I think the belt system is a well-designed system to keep students interested.

Getting my black belt was really big, it meant a great deal to me. I don't care who you are, when you start martial arts, that's in your mind—can I be a black belt? As I said before, progress in martial arts isn't about competing with other people. It's about improving yourself and challenging yourself. A black belt who is 22 years old and an incredible athlete is going to look different than a black belt who started at 50 after not exercising for 30 years.

Martial arts involves athletic ability, but it's not all about that. Grandmaster has said it himself: I don't care if someone comes in and they're super-talented, they're not going to get their black belt in six months. They have to go through the ranks and the experiences of learning everything, just like everyone else. The greatest quote about achieving black belt level is what Grandmaster said—"black belt is the beginning." It's true, because black belt isn't mastery by any means. Mastery, *maybe,* is when you get 5th *dan* (black belt rank).

Being a black belt means you have all the tools—now it's time to start building the house. The color belts are about getting the tools and accumulating them and trying to see how to use them. And by using them, I mean you start to really fine-tune yourself. You ask yourself, "okay, how do I really throw a sidekick? What part of my sidekick is not allowing me to reach my maximum power?" Now you know how to do all the techniques, it's really a matter of fine-tuning these things.

We all have habits and our bodies all work differently. You might be tighter in one leg and you start to learn that about yourself, so you know you have to give a little more on one side or a little less on the other side. You start to work on accuracy and speed. Sometimes I'll do my forms really fast just to get more of an anaerobic workout. Sometimes I'll do it more slowly to work on memorization and focus, or really work on power. You start to have a lot more control over what you're doing.

I'm a 3rd dan black belt now, and that's one of the top achievements of my life. I mean that from the bottom of my heart. I can't imagine what my life and my family's lives would've been over the last 10 years, without martial arts, and specifically without Grandmaster Kang. It's just led to so many good things and has grounded us these years. The greatest gift you can give yourself is health. You can have all the riches and fame in the world, but if you're sick and can't get better, then you can't enjoy anything.

Being a 3rd dan means a lot to me, but what's more important is that I've been here for the last 10 years and consistently dedicated myself to training regularly. Every day I exercise—I look forward to it. I find once you get grooving, you don't really have to push yourself. You're going to want to work out, you'll work out with a smile on your face. Some days you're going to be looser than others, some days things are going to feel like hard work.

I'm so grateful that my son, who was four at the time, saw the sign with Grandmaster's picture on it. Because it really set my family on a path of well-being and health, and I've made tremendous friendships in his classes. I think that mentally, martial arts is a great anti-depressant. I'm not saying that if your doctor says you need an anti-depressant, don't take it. I'm not a doctor. When I started, I was at a place where I was pretty depressed. I wasn't diagnosed by a doctor or anything, but I knew in my mind I was. And I think martial arts has really helped me deal with that. I think it can really help with depression, stress, and anxiety.

Training under Grandmaster has changed my life and my family's lives for the better. My wife and I have become Buddhists. It's been about five years now. We've been doing martial arts for ten. There's something about the focus and the way you use your mind in martial arts that led us on the path to pursue meditation and eventually brought us into studying Buddhism. It's tied into the tenets of martial arts—integrity and kindness, self-control, discipline, perseverance and dedication, and respect. Those things, if you really take them to heart, can help to start you on a spiritual path.

The fact that all five of us were doing martial arts has really kept us together as a family and instilled a lot of good habits. Look, it's easy to tell your kids to do stuff like exercise and eat right, but when you back it up by being an example, it's a lot more effective. And it's a lot easier for the kids to make it a habit when they see you doing it. As my two oldest kids grew up and began taking adult classes, it was a real pleasure for the four of us to be exercising together. That's been a real gift. It's kept the kids out of trouble. All kids anywhere can fall into destructive habits—vandalism or drugs and alcohol, we know all the possible pitfalls.

It's a community here in a way, too. There are a lot of people in the neighborhood that I know—we're parents, our kids go to the same schools. I've recommended Taekwondo to friends, I see some of them in little league and it's a sense of community. And it's a community based on health and well-being. That's something that rubs off on the kids.

One of the greatest experiences that my wife and I share with our kids is going to Taekwondo training camp in the summer, which we've done since 2003. It's just a wonderful time that we can share together. When we do the big class on the first day and there's about a hundred people there, my kids are there with us and we're all together. It's instilled some good habits and it's given them a certain foundation and structure based on really good things.

Physically, I eat better. I look better. My body's in better shape. I don't smoke anymore. I drink very moderately now. I'm a happier person. Grandmaster has played a big role in getting me there.

TESTIMONIALS

Camille Bruno

I started Grandmaster Kang's workout system in May 2006. I was 44 years old at the time. I had been looking for a new workout for a while but wasn't sure what to choose.

I have to say that for all-around fitness, this program is very effective. You get a complete workout, exercising every muscle in your body.

Training in Grandmaster Kang's system has maintained my ease of movement and flexibility. My stamina is the same, or better, than it was in my twenties. I enjoy all the activities I did when I was younger. My grandchildren don't even tire me out, try as they might!

The only obstacle I've encountered was my own mind telling me I couldn't do something when I'd never tried it. I have since learned to quiet that voice.

I'm happy I started this regimen and hope to continue for many years to come. It will be a difficult thing to stop, not only for all the physical benefits it provides, but also for the mental satisfaction that comes with it.

Joe La Rocca

Starting Grandmaster Kang's stretching exercises and food plan was a whole new way of life because I'd never really exercised before. Basically, I wasn't an active person. The only exercise I got was maybe a couple of times a year walking in the woods. So starting to seriously work out was really turning over a new leaf.

Before I started, I was somewhere around 240 pounds and fluctuating between a 42- and a 44-inch waist. I started late in life, in my fifties. It's been about two years and I'm now down to a 40-inch waist and 210–215 pounds, and it's still going.

I had no flexibility in the beginning. I was able to lift my arms but bending was a problem. First off, I hate bending. I always thought bending was a mortal sin, that's the way I looked at bending. When I bent over, I was very uncomfortable. Whatever I was trying to pick up, if I didn't get it at my first grasp, I would find myself short of breath and be red-faced when I got up.

There were days when, after a workout, I thought I would never work out again, because I thought the techniques were too hard to learn and my form was so bad. But I'm glad I didn't quit.

After a couple of months, I noticed I had a lot more flexibility and was enjoying it immensely. There was definitely weight loss and some inches off my waist. As a matter of fact, now I'm at the point where I have to buy new clothes. I have to buy smaller sizes.

My face is thinner. I now have stamina, whereas I never had stamina before! The encouragement that I receive at home from my wife and my son and Grandmaster Kang is amazing. It keeps me going. My wife loves what I'm doing for myself and what exercising has done for me—the weight loss, the decreased intake of food. I was a two cans a day of Pepsi drinker, now I'm drinking no soda at all. Maybe once in a while, if I get a craving, I'll have a can of Pepsi. Most of the time, it's seltzer.

I've also quit smoking. I'd been smoking since I was 15. I was smoking a pack-and-a-half a day, which I thought was good because when I was working, I was smoking almost three packs a day. I'm saving a lot of money now, especially living in New York with the taxes on cigarettes.

More importantly, I'm saving my life. I breathe so much easier now. It's just great, it's amazing.

Starting in my fifties, I knew I couldn't just go overboard with the exercising so I took it slowly, one day at a time. There are a lot of exercises out there, but I can't speak for any of them except for Taekwondo and stretching. What it has done for me is amazing. It's beyond my wildest dreams. Just take it a day at a time and see where it takes you. It took me very far.

Claire Jones

At 39 years old, I had aches and pains that frightened me. I was about 40 pounds overweight. I had difficulty getting up and down stairs. I was tired all the time. I knew I had to make some changes but I didn't know where to start. I was going to the gym pretty regularly and I didn't really eat very much, usually only eating one or maybe two meals a day. I felt hungry all the time, yet I was still overweight. It simply didn't make any sense to me. I thought I was doing the right things by going to the gym and eating very little, yet I still felt awful.

I started Grandmaster's program at 40. I'm 43 now and my fitness and flexibility have far exceeded what I thought was possible for me. Taekwondo will get you into shape. It focuses on good old fashioned movement. Now that I've punched through what I thought was my own ceiling, I have no reason to believe I can't become much more fit.

What has surprised me the most is not only how much flexibility I have been able to gain, but how much better stretching makes me feel. As we age it's our connective tissue that really suffers. As our connective tissue becomes less flexible, our ability to move gradually becomes limited—keeping the body supple and lubricated by exercising regularly seems to me a key way of reducing the effects of aging. For me a good workout and stretch is like having a good laugh or a cry. It just drains me of all tension—tension that, for me, leads to aches in my body.

I used to get a lot of migraines. Now I pretty much only get them when I don't eat properly, have excessive stress, and don't work out enough. I think everyone in my life would attest to the fact that, in general, I am more calm, confident, and focused. If I have something stressful or difficult I need to do, if at all possible, I try to go to a class first so I can approach it with a clear head. It has given me the confidence to try new things with my career and the drive to go after them.

As a woman who has to walk home alone at night sometimes, I realize that with a well placed front kick I could break someone's nose with the ball of my foot. It's really empowering. I have suffered, I mean really suffered, from anxiety and depression in the past. Taekwondo was the final tool that I needed to combat it effectively.

Taekwondo is about learning to relax and using tension effectively. Not only does this parallel how to be successful in many aspects of life, but I believe it permanently rewires the brain. Even when I can't get to class or I'm on vacation, I feel the effects of what I've learned.

I sit up straighter, I walk taller, and I take deep breaths when I need them. Life is better.

Gary Mirabella

Before meeting Grandmaster Kang, I was sitting on the couch doing nothing most of my days. Occasionally, I would play sports or lift some weights, but mostly, I was on that couch. My diet was terrible, it was everything you should not eat. I was drinking around 15 cups of coffee a day. When I wasn't drinking coffee, I had drinks with lots of sugar. I was smoking a pack a day.

My main goals were to lose weight and look good, and feel healthy of course. Also, to quit smoking. It took me around five months before I actually dropped the habit—it's not an easy habit to kick. I used to kill myself working out and the first thing I would do afterward is light up.

Within two to three months, I noticed a lot of mental changes. I was feeling better, standing up straighter. I had a lot more confidence. I improved my work through being more clear-minded. I had a lot more concentration.

I used to get headaches all the time before I started working out, too. I would live with headaches weeks at a time. Once the weight started coming off, the headaches were gone. No headaches ever after that. After around two months, my wife noticed I wasn't complaining about headaches anymore. I haven't gotten one since.

Around that time, there was also no pain in the mornings. My flexibility improved drastically and I was able to workout at a higher intensity with no pain the next day. I noticed also I wasn't depressed anymore, I was a lot happier. Things didn't bother me as much, I wasn't as stressed out. I was calmer, and had a more positive outlook on life.

My diet at this time was pretty good. I was eating right. I lost 50 pounds in the first three months. From there, I worked on trimming down little by little.

When I don't exercise, I have some of the old issues I used to deal with, like being stressed or anger issues. So my wife is happy that I'm calmer, more relaxed, and happier when I come home.

It's been about two years since I started exercising seriously and I'm a totally different person. I don't smoke anymore. My diet has changed. I feel like I've broken my sugar and cigarette addiction. I used to be very hot-blooded. If someone insulted me, I would immediately want to get into a fight. Now I'm the complete opposite of that, I'm very calm. People saying bad stuff doesn't bother me anymore. The furthest thing on my mind now is getting into a confrontation.

Don't give up at the first sign of pain. When you first start out, there's a lot of pain and it's very easy to give up. Once you get through the pain, you realize all the incredible things your body can do because of exercising.

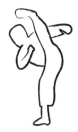

Self-Defense

Throughout the history of mankind, for whatever reason, there has always been fighting. As the most intelligent beings on this planet, we've developed ways to give ourselves an added advantage during conflicts by creating weapons, whether it is missiles, tanks, bombs, guns, or whatever else we could come up with. Even at this very moment there are researchers and scientists out there trying to create a perfect weapon, giving superiority over the rest.

If only they knew that the perfect weapon has already been created. A weapon that's armed and ready 24 hours a day, seven days a week, and doesn't need someone to control it or maintain it, because it can think for itself. And the best part is, you never have to worry about ammunition, because you can never run out of it. Are you curious to know what it is? It's us! Can you believe, yes, we are that perfect weapon. The only problem is that most of us don't realize we possess this capability. Our entire body can become a devastating weapon with the proper training.

The Eastern style of fighting was developed thousands of years ago in Asia, first as a form of mental and physical exercise, then as a tool for survival.

Nowadays, especially with the popularity of MMA (Mixed Martial Arts), I can see what all of you are thinking: two gladiators going at it in a cage. Actually, this not what martial arts is about. Martial arts is a method of "defense"—it is about understanding how to use your opponent's body to your advantage, regardless of how big they are.

But it wasn't designed by warriors or gladiators. Just the opposite—it was designed by individuals who felt they were at a disadvantage when it came to fighting. As a matter of fact, the original creators of most of these martial arts styles were barely five feet tall.

I'm not going to try to explain to you all the techniques I've practiced in the past 45 years, but I can tell you the most important concept of martial arts training: Focused energy versus dispersed energy.

Instead of giving you a long drawn-out explanation of what this means, I'm going to ask you a simple question, and I'm sure you'll figure out the answer on your own: What would do more damage, a book slammed across your face or a pencil thrusted into your eye?

I'm sure you've figured out the answer, there is no question about it—can you imagine the amount of damage a pencil stabbed into the eye can do? You're right, there's blindness, no question about it, but even worse, maybe death.

Do you see what I'm saying? Size is not a factor, but understanding how to focus your energy and striking your opponent in the most vulnerable areas of the body is the key. So something like a thumb or a finger to the eye (in place of that pencil) can be a deadly weapon.

Often, some of my new students will ask me questions about how they can defend themselves against a gun, a knife, multiple opponents, and so on. My answer to them is always that there's no way you can get out of every situation—even someone like the President, with a hundred secret service agents protecting him, can get shot. But having some knowledge of self-defense will give you an added advantage over having no knowledge at all.

Of course, there are some who will tell you that one style of martial arts is better than the others. My response to that remark is that no one style is better than the other, it's more about your personal preference and the right guidance. Really, is one ethnic group better than another? Or is one religion better than the other? You're right, there are people in the world who believe this—unfortunately, this is one of the main reasons for all the conflicts around the world, past and present.

My strong belief, as far as learning self-defense properly and effectively, is that you should participate in a martial arts program in a studio. This will give you a direct, hands-on approach and help you develop the confidence that in-home training can never do. It's not just the knowledge of the techniques, its learning to develop proper timing. Just like many things in life, timing is everything, and in a self-defense situation, how quickly and effectively you respond can be the difference between life and death. There are a lot of fine studios out there, teaching various styles of martial arts, but definitely do some research if this is the route you're seeking.

I would steer clear of any martial arts teacher who says the style he or she teaches is the best. As much as I love Taekwondo, I'm an admirer of all the martial arts and don't believe one style is superior to all the others. As for defending yourself, each one has its own pros and cons. More important than choosing a style of martial arts is finding a teacher you feel comfortable learning from.

In this self-defense section, I'm not going to teach you a defense for every offense, since no one can be a hundred percent prepared for every threat. Instead, I'm going to show you how certain parts of your body can be used as a weapon, so that whatever confrontational situation arises (hopefully none), you'll have an added advantage in defending yourself over someone with no knowledge at all.

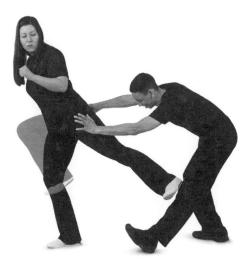

SELF-DEFENSE TECHNIQUES

Self-Defense Striking Techniques

FINGER STRIKES

Ideal for close quarters attacks where momentum can't be generated or the attacker has a size or weight advantage.

1. Attack: front choke hold
   Defense: index finger push to the base of throat

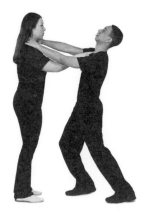

Execute in a pushing motion to the base of the throat.

2. Attack: pinned choke hold on the floor
   Defense: thumb press to the eye

Jam the thumb directly into the eyeball.

3. Attack: pinned position on the floor
   Defense: bent finger thrust to throat/windpipe

This technique is very effective, especially to the windpipe/throat area, because in addition to giving you a reach advantage, it also lets you penetrate into a narrow striking zone.

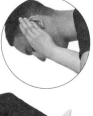

HAND STRIKES
Perfect against close attacks where your arms are free.

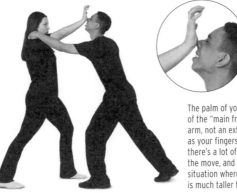

1. Attack: frontal
    assault
    Defense: palm
    thrust to the nose

The palm of your hand is part of the "main frame" of your arm, not an extension, such as your fingers. This means there's a lot of power behind the move, and it's ideal in a situation where your attacker is much taller than you.

2. Attack: side grab
    Defense: knife
    hand strike, using
    the outside edge of
    the palm with an
    open hand to
    throat/windpipe

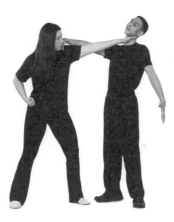

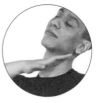

The knife hand strike is usually executed in a swinging motion using the meaty part on the side of your hand. The effectiveness of this technique is tied to its suitability for use in narrow striking areas.

3. Attack: frontal
    assault by a taller
    position
    Defense: straight
    punch to the
    groin area

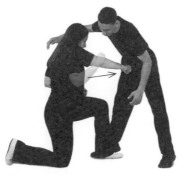

Think of a straight punch like you would the thrust of the top of a baseball bat; then think of that bat being thrust directly to the groin area.

CHAPTER 6

4. Attack: rear assault
Defense: hammer fist, using the side part of the palm with a closed hand to strike the groin area

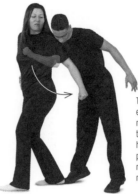

The hammer fist is executed in the same manner as a knife hand strike, the difference is that your hand is closed. So as this photo depicts, your hand movement creates a hammering motion.

JOINT STRIKES

For close attacks where more force is needed.

1. Attack: rear choke hold
Defense: elbow stab, using the tip of the elbow to the solar plexus

Joint strikes are ideal for close attacks where additional force is needed. Basically consisting of use of the knees and elbows. These areas of the body are part of the "main frame," not extensions such as your fingers or toes, which means they can be used as powerful striking tools without risk of serious injury to those areas.

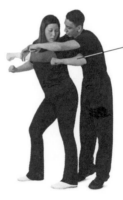

An elbow stab is executed with the pointed tip of the elbow in a thrusting motion. Very effective since all the energy is focused to one focal point.

2. Attack: close front grab
Defense: knee kick to the groin area

Standing knee kicks are most effective when executed in a forward and upward motion. If possible hold onto your attacker for added leverage.

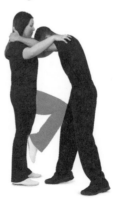

3. Attack: purse snatch
   Defense: horizontal swinging elbow hit to the face

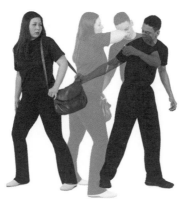

Turn toward the attacker instead of pulling away, for added momentum, while executing the horizontal elbow swing to the face.

4. Attack: frontal assault
   Defense A: Lift left arm while turning the body to the right, then smash the elbow downward on to the attacker's arm.
   Defense B: Using the same arm, hit the attacker's face with the elbow while pushing with the other hand for added power.

Defense A

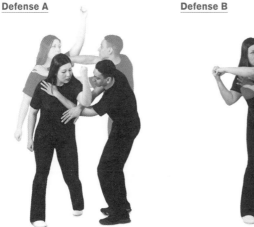

Defense B

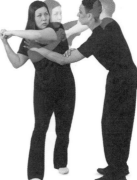

HEAD STRIKES

For situations where your arms and legs are too close to be effective.

1. Attack: hold from behind
   Defense: back of head
   strike to attacker's nose

2. Attack: front grab
   Defense: forehead smash
   to attacker's nose

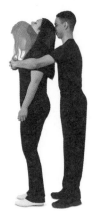

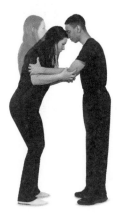

When your attacker grabs you, tilt your head forward as if looking down at the floor. (Do not lean the body forward.) Then in a rapid motion, thrust the head backward.

When the attacker grabs you, stand as tall as possible while grabbing onto his arms, then rapidly drop the top of your head down into his nose.

KICKING STRIKES

For situations where your arms are restricted or where enough distance exists between you and the attacker.

1. Attack: frontal assault
   Defense: front kick to
   attacker's groin area

2. Attack: grab from behind
   Defense: use heel to stomp
   on attacker's instep

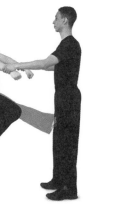

Pointing your knee to the attacker's groin area, bend your knee and then extend your leg in an upward motion.

When grabbed, lift the kicking knee up to waist level, then rapidly extend the leg downward (in a stomping motion) aiming your heel to the top of the attacker's foot.

3. Attack: front assault
   Defense: front kick to attacker's knee

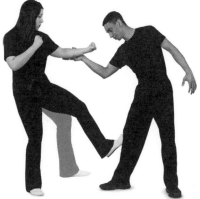

Flexing your toes back, execute a front kick to the attacker's knee, striking with the ball of your foot.

4. Attack: rear assault
   Defense: side heel kick to attacker's knee

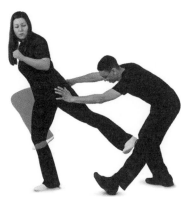

Bend the kicking leg, then extend it, aiming your heel at the front of the attacker's knee.

Conclusion

Remember, my seven week program is not a quick fix. As I've mentioned many times in this book, any fitness/diet program that guarantees quick results will take a toll on your body and your mind, and can often discourage you from continuing. Instead, it's a system designed to encourage and give you the confidence to help you understand that exercise and eating right are things you should enjoy engaging in daily for the rest of your life.

My philosophy, when it comes to health, has always been that you must take charge of it. It's your responsibility. It's the one element of life that we know that we can control, but too often we don't. I've always said to "save yourself first and be selfish" when it comes to your personal well-being, and that we're nothing without our health. No wealth, job, relationship, or whatever else that we think of as "high value" is worth anything without good health. Remember that if you're healthy, you'll have a better chance to make things happen. You'll be happier, more energetic, more focused, and a lot more positive toward life and be better able to take care of the ones you love.

Believe me, I do understand your thought process when it comes to finding time to exercise. Sometimes it's tough enough just to make it through the day. With responsibilities at work, home, parenting, relationships and whatever else that falls into your lap, life can be busy. But, then where do you come in? Who is going to tak your health, your sanity? You know the answer to that, yo cannot rely on someone else for your well-being, y charge. You only have this one body, this one life an the best of it. If we don't eat right and don't take c we're going to regret it as we age.

Be patient and know that every step you take, regardless of size, is in the right direction. Think about that baby I mentioned earlier; when they're trying to take their first steps, they might stumble or fall, but they'll still get up, because they know that walking feels a lot better than crawling.

Weight loss is one of the toughest challenges in life. Please don't give up on yourself. You must stay focused on your own progress and remember, you're not alone! Together let's stay Black Belt fit for life!